Enabling Programmable Self with HealthVault

Vaibhav Bhandari

O'REILLY®

Beijing · Cambridge · Farnham · Köln · Sebastopol · Tokyo

Enabling Programmable Self with HealthVault

by Vaibhav Bhandari

Published by O'Reilly Media, Inc., 1005 Gravenstein Highway North, Sebastopol, CA 95472.

O'Reilly books may be purchased for educational, business, or sales promotional use. Online editions are also available for most titles (*http://my.safaribooksonline.com*). For more information, contact our corporate/institutional sales department: (800) 998-9938 or *corporate@oreilly.com*.

Editor: Andy Oram	**Cover Designer:** Karen Montgomery
Production Editor: Kristen Borg	**Interior Designer:** David Futato
Proofreader: O'Reilly Production Services	**Illustrator:** Robert Romano

Revision History for the First Edition:
   2012-03-09   First release
See *http://oreilly.com/catalog/errata.csp?isbn=9781449316563* for release details.

ISBN: 978-1-449-31656-3

[LSI]

1331583495

Table of Contents

Foreword

Back in the spring of 2006, I was getting headaches consistently around lunchtime every Saturday. It was really weird. At first I didn't recognize the pattern, I just knew that my head hurt a lot, and I tried to make it go away by popping ibuprofen. The pills kind of worked, but not really. After way too long, I finally realized what must be going on.

One of the classic things everybody knows about Microsoft is that they give employees free soda. It's a pretty cool perk, but for those of us with no moderation switch, it can get a bit out of hand. When I came back to Microsoft in 2006 to start the HealthVault team, I quickly ran up a Diet Coke habit in the range of sixteen each day. All week—until Saturday, because the fridge in my house doesn't magically regenerate Diet Coke.

Suddenly it was just blindingly obvious: I was suffering from caffeine withdrawal. Now, a better man than I would have recognized that all that soda probably wasn't a good idea anyway. But instead, I just switched to caffeine-free Diet Coke and the headaches disappeared. I still spend a lot of time running to the restroom, but that's another issue altogether!

I love this story because it's so simple and obvious—and yet it offers up a clear path to making improvements in all aspects of clinical care:

- We have to *measure* our bodies over time and space.
- We have to *correlate* the data we measure to identify patterns.

Doctors measure a lot of stuff to try to understand problems in the human body: labs, imagery, vital signs, and more. But these are all done as isolated snapshots, and all too often patterns that occur over time (weeks, months, years) and space (at home, at work, traveling, etc.) hide away undiscovered.

Historically this was understandable, because measuring the body has been hard and often inconvenient. In order to be useful, the amount and diversity of data required can be significant. But the world has changed, and now it's easy for anybody to create a holistic picture of their health with data.

This is one of the big reasons we created HealthVault. We recognized the importance of a comprehensive "hub" where people could collect *all* of this diverse information together, and where smart people could provide analysis tools to look for patterns and trends. For us, the "quantified self" has been a target from day one.

Vaibhav has been part of the HealthVault team for a long time, working with partners and our internal team to constantly improve the service. He's really done a great job in this book of showing what's possible when you take a platform like HealthVault, combine it with an ecosystem of innovative measurement devices, and make the data available for analysis in familiar tools like Microsoft Excel. And that's not all—he walks us through building HealthVault apps for the web and mobile phones, somehow cramming a ton of great information into a pretty manageable read. I hope he'll inspire an avalanche of new "body hackers" who can help show us what's possible.

It's pretty amazing stuff—and frankly we've just gotten started. So have fun!

—Sean Nolan, Distinguished Engineer, Microsoft Health Solutions

Preface

Outline of the Work

Microsoft HealthVault is the most prominent example of a personally controlled health record. With its open API, flexibility, and connections with multiple health care providers, it gives people interested in monitoring their own health an unprecedented opportunity to do their own research on their own data. This concise book will explain what you can store in HealthVault, how to enable automatic updates from well-known fitness devices, and how to use programming libraries to create reports and investigate trends of interest to you. Programmable Self is a combination of Quantified Self and motivational hacks. Quantifying what you want to change about yourself and using motivational tools to ensure consistent change has been a proven recipe for successful behavioral change. It's a lot easier to start walking more if you have to tell your coworkers how many steps you walked yesterday!

Organization of This Book

Although the chapters cover different topics, they have been arranged so that the concepts and techniques in earlier chapters form a foundation for the others.

Chapter 1, Getting Started with HealthVault
> Health is critical to all of us. Health care and the infrastructure around it touch our lives and the lives of our loved ones. Many of us in pursuit of long-term health adopt goals ranging from controlling our weight to long-distance running. The health care industry is in an early stage of realizing the power of the digital world and the effectiveness of networks in helping drive change.
>
> This chapter introduces HealthVault as a powerful tool for interacting with health data. It also provides a walkthrough of functionality available to the end user through HealthVault.

Chapter 2, Quantifying Yourself

Data is a powerful tool for changing behavior. The act of simply tracking something changes one's perception of that activity. Summarizing the data over time provides a yardstick by which to measure, and the act of tracking activity over time uncovers patterns in behavior. The structured data in HealthVault provides such an opportunity. Moreover, the HealthVault ecosystem offers a variety of applications and devices to assist in this endeavor.

In this chapter we will explore how a consumer can use various devices to track critical health measures. We will also use common tools to explore the data stored by these devices into Microsoft HealthVault. We'll capture and view some data, then use a PowerShell plug-in to extract selected data to a comma-separated values (CSV) format and manipulate the data in that format.

Chapter 3, Interfacing with HealthVault

As a platform, HealthVault provides an innovative access management and programming interface for applications and devices to access a user's health information.

This chapter takes a closer look at the application programming interface (API) offered by HealthVault to enable this interaction in a programmatic fashion. We will discuss various ways in which an application or device can interface with the HealthVault platform. The code samples will use .NET interfaces because they fit well with HealthVault, but the same interfaces are available in Java, PHP, and other languages. This chapter will introduce the elements of programming that give the programmer access to data in HealthVault. Toward the end of this chapter, we will discuss various architectural options available for interfacing with HealthVault.

Chapter 4, Using the HealthVault Data Ecosystem for Self-Tracking

The Quantified Self community is engaged in enabling self-knowledge through self-tracking. Self-tracking, powered by appropriate data analysis, has been proven to trigger behavioral change. The act of self-tracking creates awareness and feedback. The hunger for, and success of, self-knowledge is evident from the growing number of self-quantifiers (currently 6,000+ in 41 cities and 14 countries).

Self-knowledge is possible only with a substantial amount of self-data. HealthVault provides more than 80 granular data types that enable tracking data regarding everything from daily exercise to genome sequences. In this chapter, we will build upon the understanding of the HealthVault API covered in Chapter 3 and extend it to develop a data-intensive self-quantifying application. Through the Quantified Self application, we will gain an understanding of HealthVault data types and application development.

Chapter 5, Enabling mHealth for Quantified Self

Having an accessible and programmable health record sets HealthVault apart. It enables a rich ecosystem of devices and mobile and web applications. Chapter 3 focused on introducing the HealthVault API, and Chapter 4 gave a good overview of HealthVault data types using a data-intensive "Quantified Self" application. This chapter takes a closer look at building mobile applications for HealthVault.

We will look at an end-to-end example of building a mood-tracking application on top of mobile platforms. This chapter will cover elements of mobile client programming using code samples for Windows Phone 7 (C#); similar interfaces are available for Android (Java) and iOS (Objective-C).

Chapter 6, The Last Mile: Releasing Applications to Users

HealthVault provides a secure and rapidly expanding platform with a rich feature set for application developers. Developer can target a wide set of users with multiple languages to enable rich functionality for Quantified Self applications.

As part of an application's life cycle, the standard steps are testing the application, releasing it to the user, and then monitoring it for anomalies. This chapter will highlight best practices for releasing, maintaining, and marketing HealthVault applications to end users.

Conventions Used in This Book

The following typographical conventions are used in this book:

Italic

Indicates new terms, URLs, email addresses, filenames, and file extensions.

`Constant width`

Used for program listings, as well as within paragraphs to refer to program elements such as variable or function names, databases, data types, environment variables, statements, and keywords.

`Constant width bold`

Shows commands or other text that should be typed literally by the user.

`Constant width italic`

Shows text that should be replaced with user-supplied values or by values determined by context.

This icon signifies a tip, suggestion, or general note.

This icon indicates a warning or caution.

Using Code Examples

This book is here to help you get your job done. In general, you may use the code in this book in your programs and documentation. You do not need to contact us for permission unless you're reproducing a significant portion of the code. For example, writing a program that uses several chunks of code from this book does not require permission. Selling or distributing a CD-ROM of examples from O'Reilly books does require permission. Answering a question by citing this book and quoting example code does not require permission. Incorporating a significant amount of example code from this book into your product's documentation does require permission.

We appreciate, but do not require, attribution. An attribution usually includes the title, author, publisher, and ISBN. For example: "*Enabling Programmable Self with Health-Vault* by Vaibhav Bhandari (O'Reilly). Copyright 2012 Vaibhav Bhandari, 978-1-449-31656-3."

If you feel your use of code examples falls outside fair use or the permission given above, feel free to contact us at *permissions@oreilly.com*.

Safari® Books Online

Safari Safari Books Online is an on-demand digital library that lets you easily search over 7,500 technology and creative reference books and videos to find the answers you need quickly.

With a subscription, you can read any page and watch any video from our library online. Read books on your cell phone and mobile devices. Access new titles before they are available for print, and get exclusive access to manuscripts in development and post feedback for the authors. Copy and paste code samples, organize your favorites, download chapters, bookmark key sections, create notes, print out pages, and benefit from tons of other time-saving features.

O'Reilly Media has uploaded this book to the Safari Books Online service. To have full digital access to this book and others on similar topics from O'Reilly and other publishers, sign up for free at *http://my.safaribooksonline.com*.

How to Contact Us

Please address comments and questions concerning this book to the publisher:

O'Reilly Media, Inc.
1005 Gravenstein Highway North
Sebastopol, CA 95472
800-998-9938 (in the United States or Canada)
707-829-0515 (international or local)
707-829-0104 (fax)

We have a web page for this book, where we list errata, examples, and any additional information. You can access this page at:

http://shop.oreilly.com/product/0636920022930.do

Community contributions, up-to-date code samples, and reusable Quantified Self spreadsheets are available at this book's companion website:

http://www.enablingprogrammableself.com

To comment or ask technical questions about this book, send email to:

bookquestions@oreilly.com

For more information about our books, courses, conferences, and news, see our website at *http://www.oreilly.com*.

Find us on Facebook: *http://facebook.com/oreilly*

Follow us on Twitter: *http://twitter.com/oreillymedia*

Watch us on YouTube: *http://www.youtube.com/oreillymedia*

Acknowledgments

Thanks to the wonderful staff at O'Reilly, especially my editor, Andy Oram, for helping me nurture the book from concept to execution. Special thanks to Fred Trotter for providing the weight data used in Chapter 1 of this book. Fred also coined the term "Programmable Self," and was gracious enough to let us use it in the book title. Thanks to Eric Friedman and the Fitbit team for helping with sleep data and the updated HealthVault integration for Fitbit.

I would like to acknowledge my family and friends for being a constant source of motivation and support. They have constantly kept up with my myriad self-experiments and projects and have pushed me to discover and learn more. I greatly acknowledge the debt they are owed, and this book is dedicated to them.

Thanks to Heidi Klinck for reviewing initial drafts and Chris Tremonte for content layout ideas. Thanks to Rob May, an exceptional developer on HealthVault team, for contributing content and code samples for the HealthVault Java library.

I am grateful to the technical reviewers for providing valuable comments on early drafts of this book, especially Rob May, Umesh Madan, Sean Nolan, Ali Emami of Microsoft, Bill Reid of Numera, and other members of HealthVault team.

Last but not least, thanks to Sean Nolan and team for conceptualizing and creating HealthVault, and Gary Wolf and team for driving the Quantified Self movement.

I hope that you will have as much fun reading this work as I did writing it, and will immerse yourself in health hacking and self-experimentation. Namaste!

CHAPTER 1

Getting Started with HealthVault

"The groundwork of all happiness is health."

—Leigh Hunt

Health is critical to all of us. Health care and the infrastructure around it touch our lives and the lives of our loved ones. Many of us in pursuit of long-term health adopt goals ranging from controlling our weight to long-distance running. The health care industry is in an early stage of realizing the power of the digital world and the effectiveness of personal health tools in helping drive change.

This chapter introduces HealthVault as a powerful tool for interacting with health data. It also provides a walkthrough of the functionality available to end users through HealthVault.

What Is HealthVault?

HealthVault is a personal data platform that allows a user to record, collect, and share all health information in a central location. A key benefit of using HealthVault is its application programming interface (API), which applications and devices can use to provide value for the end user. As depicted in Figure 1-1, HealthVault enables an ecosystem of devices and applications, with use cases ranging from tracking diet and nutrition to connecting to hospital or pharmacy systems. HealthVault currently supports more than 300 applications and 80 devices. Some devices connect to HealthVault via the HealthVault Connection Center, a complimentary client application that enables devices to upload information directly to HealthVault from a Windows PC.

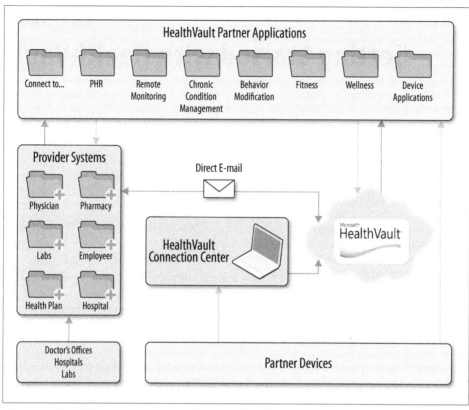

Figure 1-1. HealthVault ecosystem with devices and applications

Getting Started with HealthVault

On the HealthVault website, *http://www.healthvault.com*, a user can create an account using an existing Windows Live ID, Facebook, or OpenID account, or choose to create a new Windows Live ID. Figure 1-2 shows the sign-up screen for HealthVault.

HealthVault is currently publicly available in the United States and United Kingdom. You can create an account by entering basic demographic information and proof of human-computer interaction.

When a new user signs into HealthVault, he is greeted with a new user wizard that enables him to select tasks and allows him to connect to various services (Figure 1-3).

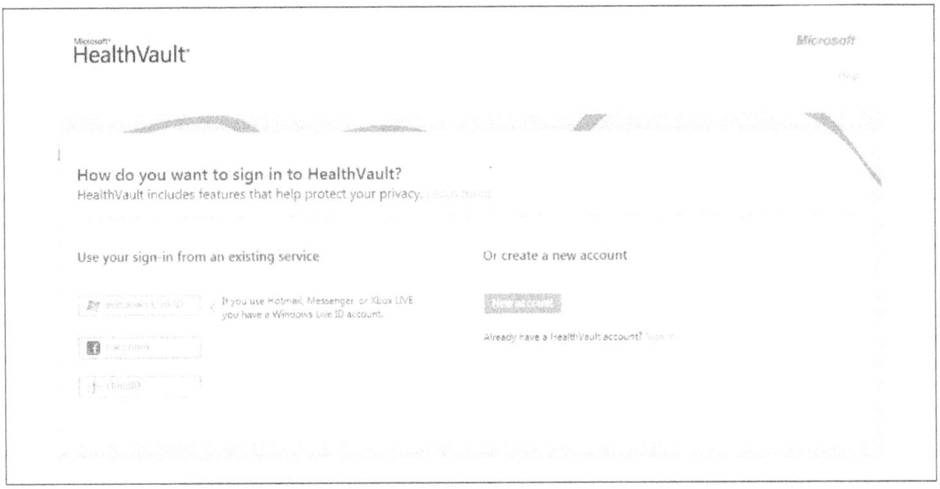

Figure 1-2. HealthVault sign-in page

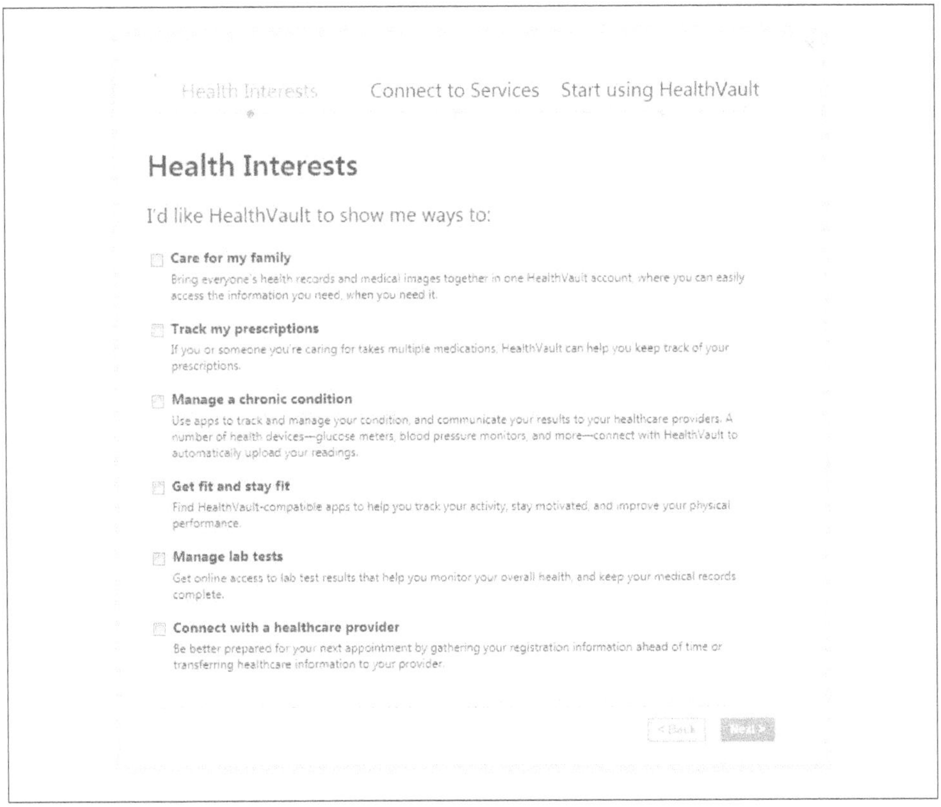

Figure 1-3. HealthVault new user wizard

Overview of HealthVault Features

This section covers a few of the most popular features in HealthVault, concentrating on ones that we'll use in this book to collect, manipulate, and share information.

Health Information

The Health Information section of the health profile provides a view of all the information in the user's health record. HealthVault supports more than 80 discrete kinds of data, from Advance Directive to Weight Goals. Through the user interface, you can edit and add health information. As Figure 1-4 indicates, you can add allergies, conditions, various measurements (blood glucose, blood pressure, peak flow, weight, height, and lab test results), files (Continuity of Care Document [CCD], Continuity of Care Record [CCR], etc.), health history (family, immunizations, procedures), and emergency provider contact information.

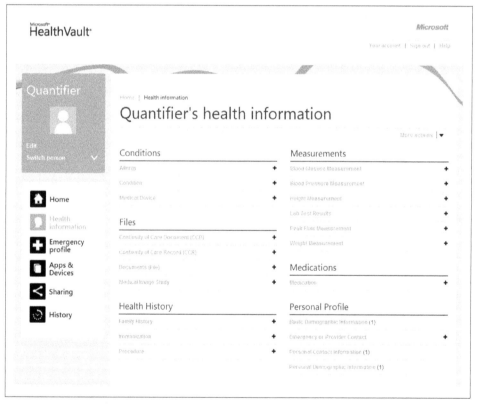

Figure 1-4. Health information input supported by HealthVault

You can also drill deeper to understand the data entered into your health profile and see the audit trail to understand how the data evolved. Figure 1-5 shows an audit history of weight in HealthVault.

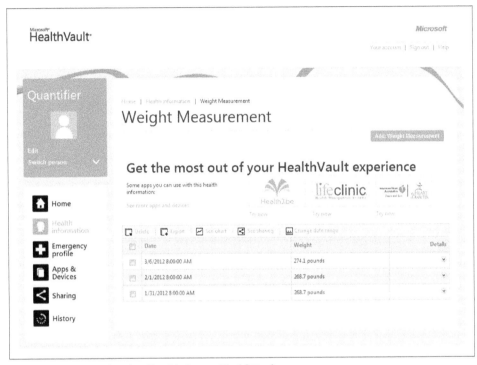

Figure 1-5. Viewing details of health data in HealthVault

Creating an Emergency Profile

Out of the box, HealthVault provides each user account with an emergency profile consisting of current allergies, conditions, medications, medical devices, and emergency contact information. A user can print, share, and update her emergency profile.

With an emergency profile, the user gets an emergency access code that could provide timely and up-to-date medical information to an emergency responder through Health-Vault.com (*http://healthvault.com*).

Figure 1-6 shows the emergency access profile. Note that in addition to printing and sharing it, a user can also access a number of HealthVault tools that provide a plethora of emergency services.

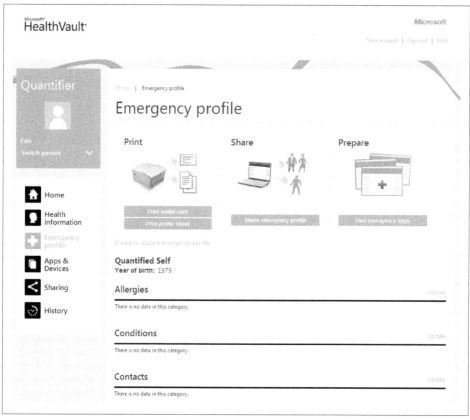

Figure 1-6. Emergency access profile

Discovering Health Tools

Using the Apps and Device section of the health profile, users can discover new applications and devices available as part of the HealthVault ecosystem. Figure 1-7 shows integrated HealthVault application and device directory. This directory is categorized by activities and conditions. A user can also get a recommended set of health tools based on their preferences set in the new user wizard (Figure 1-3). This searchable directory functionality was recently added to HealthVault.

Through this section, users can also review and revoke access permissions to all the HealthVault applications they have used over time.

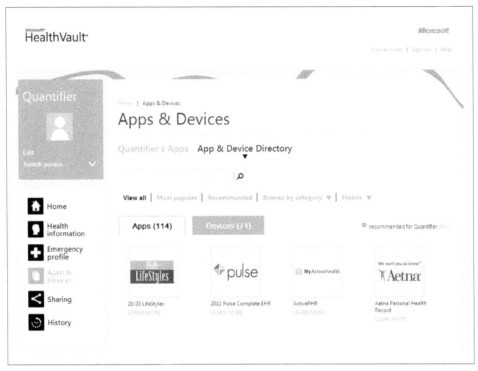

Figure 1-7. Discovering HealthVault applications and devices

Sharing

Using the Sharing section of the health profile, users can view with whom and how this information is being shared. Users can invite people to view granular information in their health profiles. The data used in this book was collected from gracious contributors by using this sharing functionality for specific types of health data. As Figure 1-8 shows, through the Sharing pane, users can review and revoke access to other people.

History

Having a granularly shareable health profile enables a plethora of care coordination scenarios. However, we do want to know how and when our sensitive health information is being accessed and updated. As Figure 1-9 shows, through the History pane of the health profile, users can view the ways their health information has been accessed. I frequently look at the "Changes made in last 30 days" and review who has accessed and updated my record.

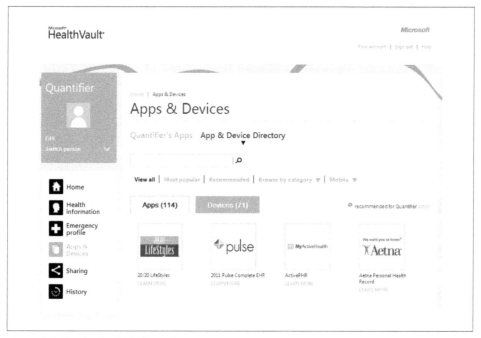

Figure 1-8. Sharing health information

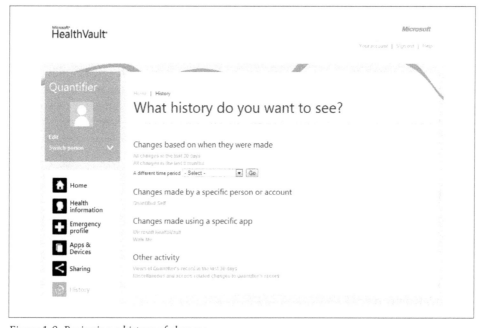

Figure 1-9. Reviewing a history of changes

Working with Health Data

Data is a powerful tool to understand behaviors and trigger appropriate, measured change. Users can find out interesting trends by running calculations on their data stored in HealthVault, as I'll show throughout this book.

For instance, through the health information section, a user can chart his weight readings (Figure 1-10).

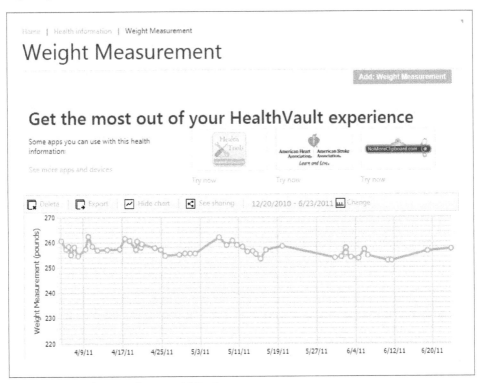

Figure 1-10. Tracking weight in HealthVault

You will see that over the last several readings, weight has been stable around 257 pounds. Nonetheless, I would like to take this a bit further and analyze these readings. To do this, I click on the Export button in the health information section. This gives me the readings in a comma-separated values (CSV) format, which I can then open in Microsoft Excel or any spreadsheet program (Figure 1-11). If you don't have weight data, I encourage you to download the sample spreadsheet with weight data included as part of this book's examples and follow along with that data.

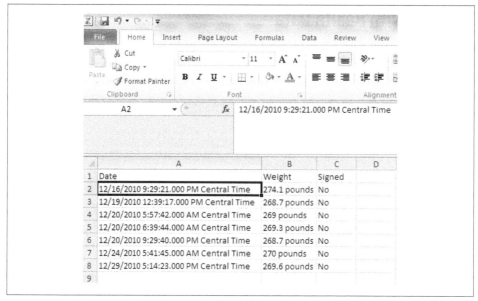

Figure 1-11. Weight readings in Microsoft Excel

Using Excel, I can clean the data so I can chart and analyze it further. I can add a series date attribute by just using the date from the first column (Figure 1-12).

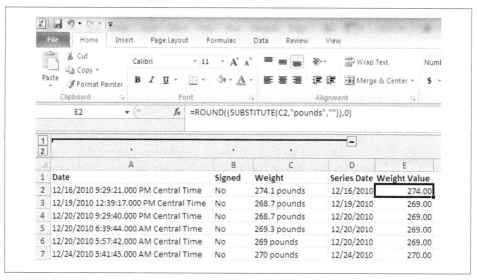

Figure 1-12. Using Excel to clean up the date

The formula DATEVALUE(LEFT(A2, FIND("")), A2))) converts the cell to a date value by picking the left side of the date format before the first space in column A2. The formula ROUND(SUBSTITUTE(C2, "pounds")),0) removes the pound unit in column C and rounds the value to the nearest integer.

Using Excel, I can find the average weight over the last set of readings and in fact plot my weight over a number of months to uncover the monthly trend (Figure 1-13).

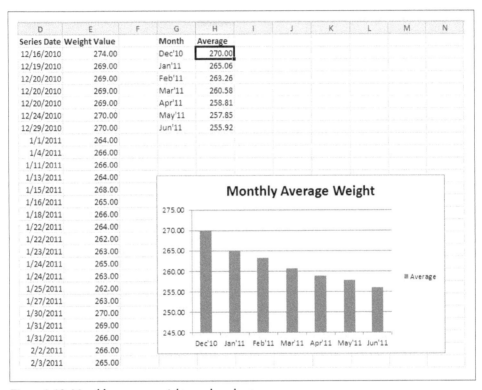

Figure 1-13. Monthly average weight as a bar chart

Managing weight is only one scenario where you can use health tools to gain insights. This book's associated website, *http://enablingprogrammableself.com*, has a repository of spreadsheets that can give you inspiration for additional care scenarios.

Using Partner Applications

So far, we have looked at the mechanisms provided within HealthVault to track, update, and visualize health information. Outside applications, however, offer even more information. For instance, the Mayo Clinic Health Manager application (*https://health manager.mayoclinic.com*) can track your weight toward an intended goal (Figure 1-14).

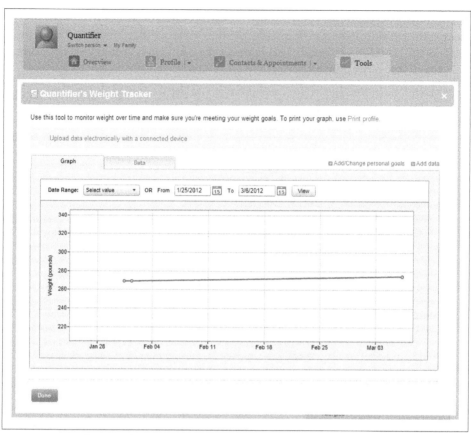

Figure 1-14. Tracking weight against a goal

The Mayo Clinic Health Manager is able to access all the weight information from a user's HealthVault account using the HealthVault API. If you're not a programmer, you can benefit from many such applications that add value to HealthVault by allowing you to track and measure health data. If, however, you have modest programming skills in almost any modern language, this book will show how you can create your own.

The HealthVault .NET Web SDK provides an abstraction on HealthVault APIs to simplify working with the platform. Example 1-1 is a .NET program that uses the SDK to extract all the weights from a user's HealthVault record into a dictionary.

Example 1-1. Accessing HealthVault through the .NET Web SDK to read weight measurements

```
using System;
using System.Collections.Generic;

using System.Web;
```

```
using Microsoft.Health;
using Microsoft.Health.Web;
using Microsoft.Health.ItemTypes;
using Microsoft.Health;

public partial class HelloWorldPage : HealthServicePage
{
    protected void Page_Load(object sender, EventArgs e)
    {

        HealthRecordSearcher searcher = PersonInfo.SelectedRecord.CreateSearcher();

        HealthRecordFilter filter = new HealthRecordFilter(Weight.TypeId);
        searcher.Filters.Add(filter);

        HealthRecordItemCollection items = searcher.GetMatchingItems()[0]; ❶

        Dictionary<string, string> weights = new Dictionary<string, string>();

        foreach (Weight item in items)
        {
            weights[item.When.ToString()] = item.Value.ToString();
        }

        WeightView.DataSource = weights;
        WeightView.DataBind();
    }
}
```

The steps in extracting data are: create a searcher, add a filter to restrict the output to the field or rows you want, and then run a search. `searcher.GetMatchingItems()` in line ❶ of Example 1-1 actually issues a HealthVault GetThings API request with a query configured to fetch all the `Weight` items from the user'ss HealthVault record. We will learn more about the API and account management in Chapter 3, and more about the data types in Chapter 4.

In the next chapter, we will delve deeper into the HealthVault device and application ecosystem.

CHAPTER 2

Quantifying Yourself

"If you cannot measure it, you cannot improve it."

—Lord Kelvin

Data is a powerful tool for changing behavior. The act of simply tracking changes one's perception of that activity. Summarizing the data over time provides a yardstick by which to measure, and the act of tracking activity over time uncovers patterns in behavior and provides definitive answers to self-experimentation questions. The structured data in HealthVault provides such an opportunity. Moreover, the HealthVault ecosystem offers a variety of applications and devices to assist in this endeavor.

In this chapter we will explore how a consumer can use various devices to track critical health measures. We will also use common tools to explore the data stored by devices in Microsoft HealthVault. We'll capture and view some data, then use a PowerShell plug-in to extract selected data to a CSV format and manipulate the data in that format.

Fitbit is being used in this chapter just to illustrate the ways you can use data from all kinds of devices, so long as they provide a gateway to HealthVault. If you're not using Fitbit, I encourage you to download the sample Fitbit sleep data included as part of this book's examples, and follow along.

How Fitbit Tracks Sleep

Fitbit is a pedometer on steroids that enables you to monitor a number of aspects of daily living. This chapter concentrates on sleep because Fitbit has been very popular with users trying to understand and change their sleep patterns. Fitbit provides an arm band (Figure 2-1) that tracks whether you're awake or asleep based on your activity level. Alternatively, users can select an on/off mode to indicate whether they're asleep.

Fitbit also provides a base station that wirelessly uploads information from the device to the Fitbit web service. Not having to worry about uploading information is a great value-add provided by this product.

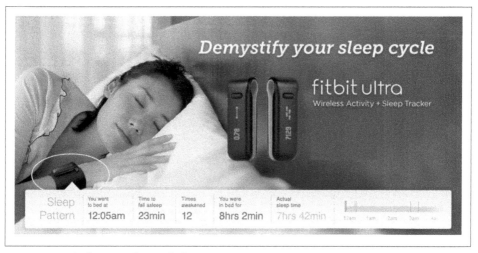

Figure 2-1. Fitbit being used to track sleep

Sending Data to HealthVault

Fitbit enables users to sync their data automatically with HealthVault. Once you have a Fitbit account, you can choose the "Share stats" page (Figure 2-2), which becomes available after clicking on the account settings.

The "Share stats" page, among other services, enables a link to HealthVault (Figure 2-3).

Any application connecting to HealthVault has to get consent from the user for the kinds of data it will be reading from or writing to Microsoft HealthVault. The user control is a two-step process. In the first step, the user chooses the context of the record being authorized (Figure 2-4). As Figure 2-4 shows, in my case I have the option of using the application for my record or my mother's. In the second step, the user grants access to the specific health data being shared with the application (Figure 2-5). As Figure 2-5 shows, the Fitbit application wants to access to my Exercise, Sleep Session, and other health information. We will learn in more detail about the user authentication and authorization system in Chapter 3.

Clicking on the "Information that Fitbit needs to be able to access to work as intended," you will notice that Fitbit wants to access a user's Custom Data, Fitness, Measurements, and Personal Profile, as shown in Figure 2-6. In the line below the heading you will notice Application-Specific Information, Exercise, Sleep Session, Personal Contact Information, and Personal Demographic Information, which are granular HealthVault data types. HealthVault has about 80+ granular data types that form the building blocks for various kinds of health information (Fitness, Measurement, etc.). The data types are optimized to work with different devices and health systems. We will learn more about HealthVault data types and vocabularies in Chapter 4.

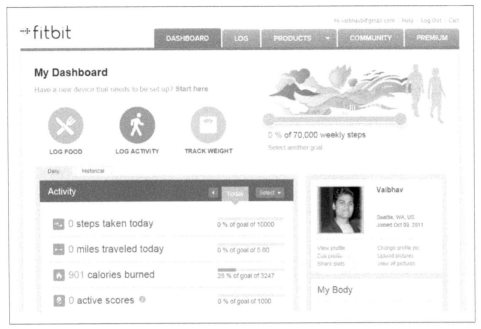

Figure 2-2. Fitbit "Share stats" feature

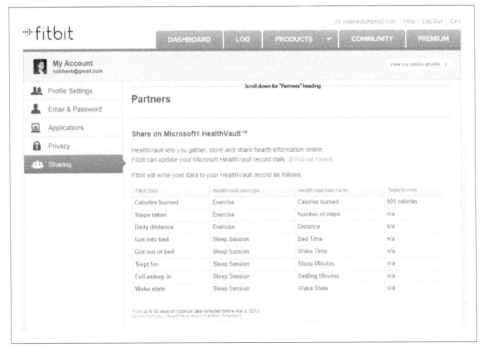

Figure 2-3. Connecting Fitbit with Microsoft HealthVault

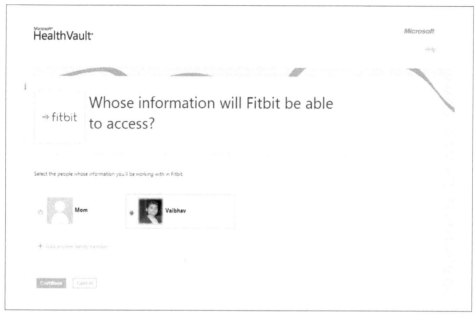

Figure 2-4. Choosing the context of a HealthVault record to work with an application

Understanding the Data Model

Fitbit collects pedometer and sleep data. When the device syncs its data to Health-Vault's granular types, it stores data as detailed in Table 2-1.

Table 2-1. Fitbit HealthVault data mapping

Fitbit data	HealthVault data type	HealthVault field name
Calories Burned	Exercise	Calories burned
Steps Taken	Exercise	Number of steps
Daily Distance	Exercise	Distance
Got in to bed	Sleep Session	Bed Time
Got out of bed	Sleep Session	Wake Time
Slept for	Sleep Session	Sleep Minutes
Fell asleep in	Sleep Session	Settling Minutes
Wake State	Sleep Session	Wake State

As a user, we are interested in tracking all the information about sleep as collected by Fitbit. As you will note from Table 2-1, we should look at the HealthVault Sleep Session data type for tracking sleep and the HealthVault Exercise data type for tracking Fitbit pedometer data.

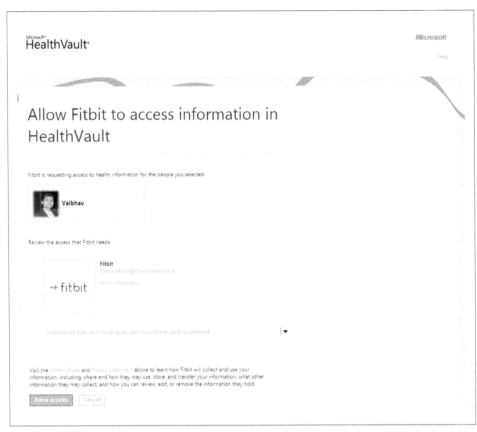

Figure 2-5. *Authorizing an application to access a user's health data*

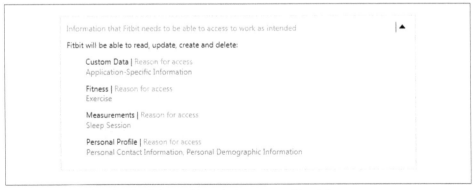

Figure 2-6. *Granular details of the HealthVault data accessed by Fitbit*

Exploring the HealthVault Data

You can look at the data stored from Fitbit in the HealthVault user interface (sometimes referred to as the HealthVault Shell), as shown in Figure 2-7.

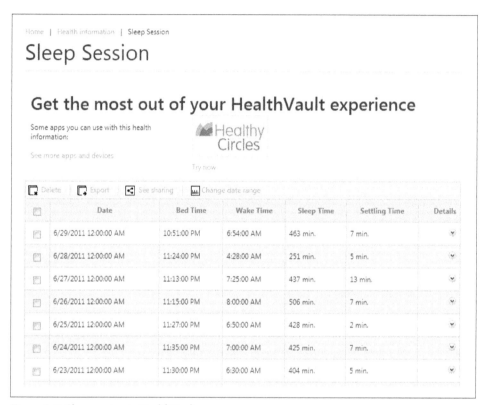

Figure 2-7. Sleep session in HealthVault

Viewing information through the HealthVault user interface is convenient, but a user cannot retrieve the entire information by exporting the data. As a power user and a quantifier, I would like the data to be available to me to do some data-noodling. For that purpose, I would get this data in command-line format using the HealthVault PowerShell plug-in (HvPosh). You can find the details of installing and extending this plug-in at *https://github.com/vaibhavb/HvPosh*. PowerShell can export data to a standard CSV format that can be consumed by a variety of other tools, simple or advanced, that let you do calculations and generate charts.

Once you have installed PowerShell, load HealthVault's plug-in into Windows PowerShell using:

```
Powershell> import-module HvPosh
```

Then, grant access to HealthVault PowerShell interface using the following command line. Note that this command will walk you through the same record-picking interface and authentication and authorization interface as we used earlier for the Fitbit application:

```
Powershell> Grant-HVPermission
```

Once you have access to HealthVault within PowerShell, you can start using the utility from the command line and extract information pertinent to Sleep Session:

```
Powershell> Get-Things -item Sleep-Session | format-table
```

The results for my sample data are shown in Figure 2-8.

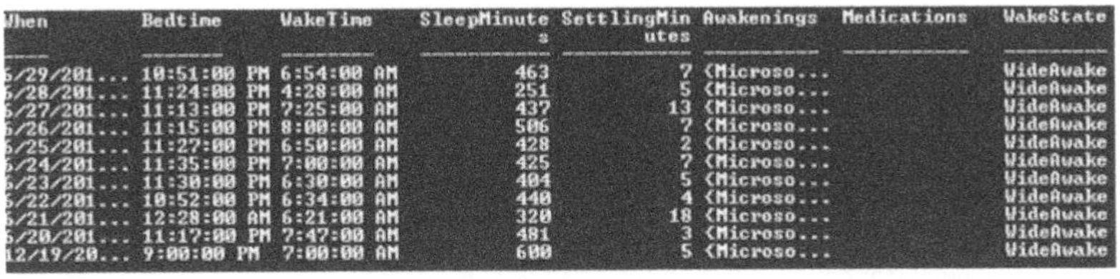

When	Bedtime	WakeTime	SleepMinutes	SettlingMinutes	Awakenings	Medications	WakeState
6/29/201...	10:51:00 PM	6:54:00 AM	463	7	{Microso...		WideAwake
6/28/201...	11:24:00 PM	4:28:00 AM	251	5	{Microso...		WideAwake
6/27/201...	11:13:00 PM	7:25:00 AM	437	13	{Microso...		WideAwake
6/26/201...	11:15:00 PM	8:00:00 AM	506	7	{Microso...		WideAwake
6/25/201...	11:27:00 PM	6:50:00 AM	428	2	{Microso...		WideAwake
6/24/201...	11:35:00 PM	7:00:00 AM	425	7	{Microso...		WideAwake
6/23/201...	11:30:00 PM	6:30:00 AM	404	5	{Microso...		WideAwake
6/22/201...	10:52:00 PM	6:34:00 AM	440	4	{Microso...		WideAwake
6/21/201...	12:28:00 AM	6:21:00 AM	320	18	{Microso...		WideAwake
6/20/201...	11:17:00 PM	7:47:00 AM	481	3	{Microso...		WideAwake
12/19/20...	9:00:00 PM	7:00:00 AM	600	5	{Microso...		WideAwake

Figure 2-8. Structured data from Sleep Session as retrieved by PowerShell

If you don't have a Fitbit and want to follow along, you can import data from the file *Sleep-Data.xml* available in the code associated with Chapter 3. Following is the command to import this data:

```
Powershell> Import-HvDataXml -File Sleep-Data.xml
```

You can understand the data further by exploring the individual properties. Figure 2-9 shows how you can select particular properties of a HealthVault data type using the PowerShell `select-object` command:

```
Powershell> get-things sleep | select-object When, Bedtime, WakeTime | format-table
```

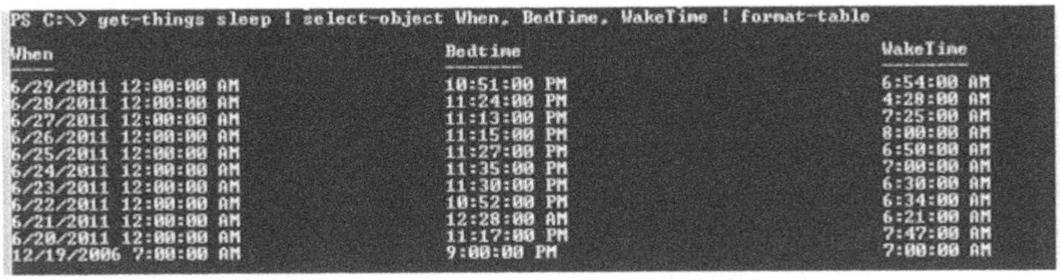

```
PS C:\> get-things sleep | select-object When, BedTime, WakeTime | format-table

When                    Bedtime         WakeTime
----                    -------         --------
6/29/2011 12:00:00 AM   10:51:00 PM     6:54:00 AM
6/28/2011 12:00:00 AM   11:24:00 PM     4:28:00 AM
6/27/2011 12:00:00 AM   11:13:00 PM     7:25:00 AM
6/26/2011 12:00:00 AM   11:15:00 PM     8:00:00 AM
6/25/2011 12:00:00 AM   11:27:00 PM     6:50:00 AM
6/24/2011 12:00:00 AM   11:35:00 PM     7:00:00 AM
6/23/2011 12:00:00 AM   11:30:00 PM     6:30:00 AM
6/22/2011 12:00:00 AM   10:52:00 PM     6:34:00 AM
6/21/2011 12:00:00 AM   12:28:00 AM     6:21:00 AM
6/20/2011 12:00:00 AM   11:17:00 PM     7:47:00 AM
12/19/2006 7:00:00 AM   9:00:00 PM      7:00:00 AM
```

Figure 2-9. Three columns of structured data from Sleep Session as retrieved by PowerShell

In fact, I want to be able to explore details of awakenings. This is particularly relevant for learning about patterns of sleep disturbances. Figure 2-10 shows the output from the following command:

```
Powershell> get-things sleep | select-object -expandproperty Awakenings | format-table
```

```
PS C:\> get-things sleep | select-object  -expandproperty Awakenings | format-table

When
----
3:00:00 AM
3:00:00 AM
3:00:00 AM
3:00:00 AM
3:00:00 AM
3:00:00 AM
3:00:00 AM
3:00:00 AM
3:00:00 AM
3:00:00 AM
9:00:00 PM
```

Figure 2-10. Understanding the pattern of Awakenings

Now you can enable some data crunching by exporting this data to a CSV file and switching the data analysis to Microsoft Excel or Google Spreadsheets:

```
Powershell> get-things sleep | select-object When, SleepMinutes, SettlingMinutes |
export-csv SleepData.csv
```

This creates the file *SleepData.csv* with the selected data.

Analyzing the HealthVault Data

Once you have all the data in CSV file, you can open it in Excel (Figure 2-11) and analyze sleep patterns. You will notice that the spreadsheet has data for each sleep session specifying when that session occurred, the total sleep time in minutes, and the time it took to get to bed, termed as `SettlingMinutes`. I want to understand this data better, so I create a sleep pattern X-Y scatter plot for this information (Figure 2-14).

	A	B	C	D
1	#TYPE Selected.Microsoft.Health.ItemTypes.SleepJournalAM			
2	When	SleepMinutes	SettlingMinutes	
3	6/29/2011 0:00	463	7	
4	6/28/2011 0:00	251	13	
5	6/27/2011 0:00	437	5	
6	6/26/2011 0:00	506	7	
7	6/25/2011 0:00	428	2	
8	6/24/2011 0:00	425	7	
9	6/23/2011 0:00	404	5	
10	6/22/2011 0:00	440	4	
11	6/21/2011 0:00	320	18	
12	6/20/2011 0:00	481	3	
13	12/19/2006 7:00	600	5	

Figure 2-11. Sleep session data in an Excel spreadsheet

As Figure 2-12 reveals, for the duration of this week the median sleep has been around 400 minutes (i.e., around 6.5 hours), and as the data clearly shows, for the days when it took the longest to get to sleep, the duration of sleep has been lower. So a good indicator of not been able to get to sleep in 10 minutes is a lower and poorer quality of sleep.

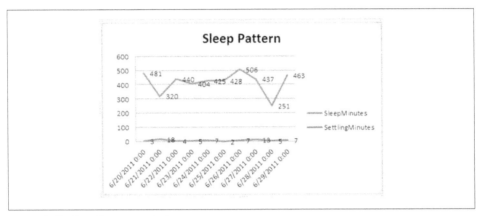

Figure 2-12. Sleep Pattern analysis

In fact, for this duration I also want to understand the patterns around awakenings. So using PowerShell we generate another CSV file that focuses on awakenings:

```
Powershell> get-things sleep | select-object effectivedate -expandproperty awakenings | Export-Csv d:\sleep-date-aw.csv
```

We can open the file in Excel and visualize how the awakenings are triggered. It's very obvious that most awakenings are for a duration of 10 minutes around 3 a.m, as shown in Figure 2-13. I know that this is because the workshop in my neighborhood is doing an early project and the noise around that time wakes me up.

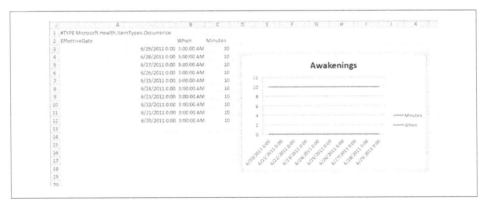

Figure 2-13. Awakenings pattern analysis

We can even take it a step further and correlate the sleep information with other types of data. Fitbit also contains activity data, and we can try to associate the pedometer information with the existing sleep data.

Using the PowerShell HealthVault plug-in, we can grab the appropriate fitness data from HealthVault:

```
Powershell> Get-Things exercise | where-object {$_.Activity.Name -eq "walk"} |
    select-object
-expandproperty Activity | export-csv pedometer.csv
```

Adding the pedometer data to what we obtained in Figure 2-12 gives us a way to correlate physical activity to sleep, as shown in Figure 2-14.

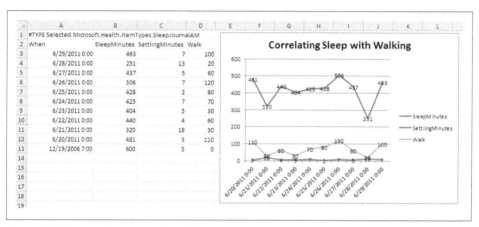

Figure 2-14. Correlating sleep with walking exercise

Note that we scaled the steps information from the pedometer by dividing it by 100, so it would play nice on the graph . Using this information, one can say it's possible that the days on which you got less sleep were due to lack of exercise—but on the other hand, the settling time was high on those days as well. So maybe as a behavioral change, one can resolve to walk at least 5,000 steps to ensure a good sleep.

This might change in the long run, but that is the joy of learning from data and motivating a behavior shift! This book's associated website, *http://enablingprogrammable self.com*, has a repository of spreadsheets that can inspire additional self-experimentation scenarios. You are invited to participate in the community and contribute self-tracking spreadsheets that you have found useful.

In upcoming chapters, we will learn how we can automate some of the work we have done in this chapter with the HealthVault application programming interface.

CHAPTER 3

Interfacing with HealthVault

"Things would have changed if I had timely access to
electronic medical records."

—Regina Holliday

As a platform, HealthVault provides an innovative access management and programming interfaces for applications and devices to access a user's health information.

In the previous chapter we discovered how to fetch and manipulate data stored in HealthVault. This chapter takes a closer look at the API offered by HealthVault to enable this interaction in a programmatic fashion. We will discuss various ways in which an application or device can interface with the HealthVault platform. The code samples will use .NET interfaces because they fit well with HealthVault, but the same interfaces are available in Java, PHP, and other languages. The chapter will introduce the elements of programming that give the programmer access to data in HealthVault. Toward the end of this chapter, we will discuss various architectural options available for interfacing an application or device with HealthVault. We'll start by discussing accounts because the first task is to get access to your own account.

Accounts and Records

HealthVault provides innovative access management to let a family health manager access and manage the records of various family members. Mom, serving as the family health manager, can create records for her husband and children. In Figure 3-1, Jane has created accounts for her husband, Tom, and two kids, Chris and Sara. She has full access to all information in her family's HealthVault records.

Additionally, HealthVault enables the same records to be accessed through multiple accounts. Full access can be thought of as custodial access to the record. In Figure 3-2, Jane has full access to her family's health information. Tom has also signed up to share the responsibility of managing the health information of their kids, Chris and Sara, and also has full access to their health information.

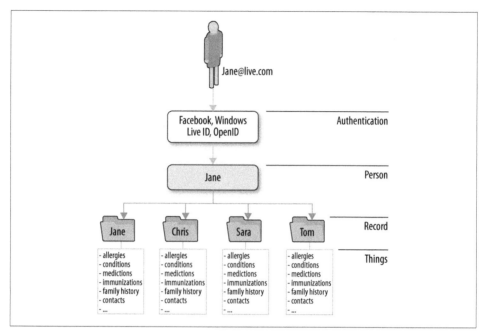

Figure 3-1. Multiple records under one HealthVault account

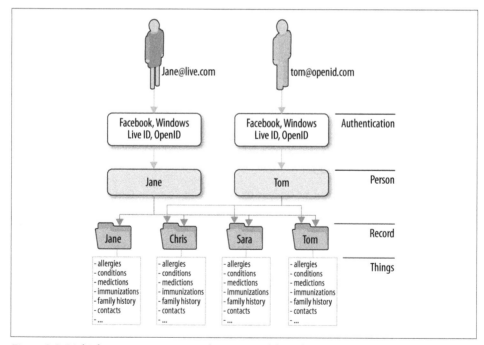

Figure 3-2. Multiple accounts pointing to the same HealthVault records

Account Information

An application gets access to HealthVault account information through an API called Get-PersonInfo. This API returns a structure called PersonInfo, which in turn consists of the records associated with a HealthVault account (Example 3-1).

Example 3-1. PersonInfo data structure

```
PS C:\Windows\system32> Get-Personinfo

PersonId              : 0ce0d6e0-cfaf-4464-abea-6d0253078df6
Name                  : Vaibhav Bhandari
ApplicationSettings   :
SelectedRecord        : Vaibhav Bhandari
AuthorizedRecords     : {[b11511c8-c30d-4ffd-8d98-f433d0b5827b, Vaibhav Bhandari]}
PreferredCulture      : en-US
PreferredUICulture    : en-US
Connection            :
ApplicationConnection : Microsoft.Health.HealthClientAuthorizedConnection
```

Using the HealthVault PowerShell plug-in, you can try out the Get-PersonInfo API using the command `get-personinfo`. The structure returned consists of a unique `PersonId` for the account and a set of record identifiers authorized to be used with the application for this particular account. Any pertinent information for the application is stored in `ApplicationSettings`. The user's preferred language and display settings are stored in the `PreferredCulture` and `PreferredUICulture` fields, respectively.

An application can decide to work with only one record at a time, termed as a *single record application* (SRA), or provide an interface to work with multiple records associated with the signed-in user, termed as a *multiple record application* (MRA). "Interfacing with HealthVault" on page 46 describes how to enable each of these record management capabilities in detail.

HealthVault Application Programming Interface

A HealthVault application interacts with two distinct resources:

- The HealthVault Platform (*https://platform.healthvault.com/platform/wildcat .ashx*)
- The HealthVault Shell (*https://account.healthvault.com*).

The HealthVault Platform provides XML over HTTP requests to manipulate data hosted by the service, and the HealthVault Shell provides account management, user authentication, and other services.

HealthVault provides a development environment for partners to develop their applications. The development environment is hosted at *https://platform.healthvault-ppe .com/latform* for the HealthVault Platform and *https://account.healthvault-ppe.com* for the HealthVault Shell.

Each HealthVault application gets a unique identifier called an AppID. Developers can get a free application identifier using the HealthVault Configuration Center (*https://config.healthvault-ppe.com*).

 For our example application, we are using an application ID that was already created for a HelloWorld sample application. In Chapter 4, we will create our own application.

HealthVault Shell Interface

The HealthVault Shell provides its functionality primarily by redirecting the end user's browser. The HealthVault Shell presents a secure user interface dialog in the browser. These dialogs help with user authentication, authorization, record selection, and managing the user's experience around health data.

An application communicates its intention to the HealthVault Shell using a URI construct like *https://account.healthvault.com/redirect.aspx?target=<ShellTarget>&targetqs=<ShellTargetParams>*.

The *<ShellTarget>* parameter specifies the intent of the application, which could range from prompting the user to authorize the application to letting the user view their health items. Table 3-1 summarizes some of these targets; a detailed list of the Shell Targets is available on the HealthVault MSDN at *http://msdn.microsoft.com/en-us/library/ff803620.aspx*.

Table 3-1. HealthVault Shell redirect interface (partial list)

HealthVault Shell Target	Purpose
AUTH	Prompts the user to authorize himself and select record(s) to be used with an application
APPREDIRECT	Redirects a user to another HealthVault application
CREATEACCOUNT	Allows an application to create a new HealthVault account, and redirects to the application after account authorization
CREATEAPPLICATION	Enables a client or desktop application to create an instance of its application on the device
RECONCILE	Enables an application to redirect to the HealthVault Shell for reconciling a CCR/CCD with a user record
VIEWITEMS	Allows an application to redirect a user to view or create health record items using the HealthVault Shell

In certain circumstances, the HealthVault Shell needs to communicate with the application. For example, if a user wants to know the privacy statement of the application or if the user decides to not authorize permission for the application to access their health items, the HealthVault shell would then need to communicate with the application. HealthVault requires applications to register a "Redirect URL" for the functionality they provide. The Redirect URL should be a secure (HTTPS) URL that can respond to a request of this nature:

> *https://<ApplicationRedirectURL>?target=<ApplicationTarget>&targetqs=<ApplicationTargetParameters>*

The *<ApplicationTarget>* specifies the desired action to get serviced; it could range from the user asking for a privacy statement to the user rejecting the application's authorization request. Table 3-2 summarizes some of these targets; a detailed list of the Application Targets is available at *http://msdn.microsoft.com/en-us/library/ff803620 .aspx.*

Table 3-2. HealthVault Application Targets (partial list)

HealthVault Application Target	Purpose
APPAUTHSUCCESS	Notifies the application that the user successfully logged in and/or granted authorization to the application.
SIGNOUT	Notifies the application that the user logged out of her HealthVault session. The application can then do cleanup and show a sign-out page.
SELECTEDRECORD CHANGED	Notifies the application that the user successfully changed the selected record. "Record Management: Diving Deep" on page 41 shows example of handling this.
PRIVACY	Notifies the application that the user wants to view her privacy statement.
SERVICEAGREEMENT	Notifies the application that the user wants to view its terms of use or service agreement.

HealthVault Platform APIs

The HealthVault Platform provides a number of APIs to enable access to application and user data; these APIs are well documented at *http://developer.healthvault.com/pa ges/methods/methods.aspx*. The following discussion will focus on the kinds of functionality provided by these APIs. Table 3-3 summarizes the APIs available from the HealthVault platform.

Table 3-3. HealthVault API summary

HealthVault API category	API names	Purpose
Authentication	CreateAuthenticatedSessionToken	Authenticate an application and a user.
	RemoveApplicationRecordAuthorization	
	NewApplicationCreationInfo	
	NewSignupCode	
	GetPersonInfo	
	GetAuthorizedRecords	

HealthVault API category	API names	Purpose
Reading Health Items	GetThings	A rich interface to retrieve health items along with an associated digital signature or streamed BLOBs.
Adding & Updating Health Items	PutThings	Enable an application to add or update health item data.
	OverwriteThings	
	BeginPutBlob	
Delete Health Items	RemoveThings	Enables an application to delete data.
Patient Connect	AssociatePackageId	Enable clinical applications to create a temporary drop-off or permanent connection for consumers without having a web interface.
	BeginPutConnectPackageBlob	
	CreateConnectPackage	
	CreateConnectRequest	
	GetAuthorizedConnectRequests	
	DeletePendingConnectPackage	
	DeletePendingConnectRequest	
Asynchronous Processing	GetAuthorizedPeople	Enable an application to work asynchronously with HealthVault and create a publish/subscribe model.
	GetUpdatedRecordsForApplication	
	GetEventSubscriptions	
	UpdateEventSubscription	
	SubscribeToEvent	
	UnsubscribeToEvent	
Messaging	SendInsecureMessage	Enable applications to send messages to consumers using these APIs.
	SendInsecureMessageFromApplication	
Terminology	GetVocabulary	Enable applications to retrieve or search terminologies hosted by HealthVault.
	SearchVocabulary	
Application Management	SetApplicationSettings	Enable an application to store a record-specific setting and manage derivative applications.
	GetApplicationSettings	
	AddApplication	
	UpdateApplication	
Service Discovery	GetServiceDefinition	Help with service discovery.
	GetThingType	
OpenQuery	SaveOpenQuery	These are hardly used, but they give the ability to run pre-canned queries for a health record.
	GetOpenQueryInfo	
	DeleteOpenQuery	

Authentication and authorization APIs

Applications authenticate themselves to the HealthVault platform using the CreateAuthenticatedSessionToken API. Users are authenticated through HealthVault.com (*http://healthvault.com*), and applications can get tokens for authorization using the HealthVault Shell redirect interface at *http://msdn.microsoft.com/en-us/library/ff803620.aspx*.

CreateAuthenticatedSessionToken, or CAST, is the most commonly used HealthVault API. This API provides authentication tokens for clients as well as web applications. Most HealthVault wrappers provide an API for this purpose.

Individual methods are available for an application to fetch record and person authorization details. Most notably, NewApplicationCreationInfo is used by mobile clients to receive security keys from the HealthVault platform.

Reading health items

The core function that lets an application read items from a user's HealthVault record is GetThings. We will discuss this API in detail in "GetThings" on page 35, but to summarize, this API provides the ability to query HealthVault, fetch a health item with granular details, and fetch large BLOB items, such as images.

After CreateAuthenticatedSessionToken, GetThings is the most commonly used HealthVault API.

Creating and updating health items

The counterpart of GetThings is PutThings. It is used by most applications to update and create health items. We will discuss this function in detail in the section "PutThings" on page 39.

OverwriteThings allows applications to force overwrites on existing health items. This API generally is not used.

HealthVault, unlike most personal health platforms, provides a mechanism to store large files such as medical images. Applications can upload large chunks of information by using the BeginPutBlob API. It is fairly tricky to use, but there is good documentation on how to use it via raw XML interfaces at *http://msdn.microsoft.com/en-us/library/ff803584.aspx*, as well as through the HealthVault .NET SDK at *http://msdn.microsoft.com/en-us/library/ff803576.aspx*.

Deleting health items

DeleteThings is the one of the simplest HealthVault functions, allowing applications to delete individual health items from a user's record. HealthVault keeps an audit trail of all operations, including the delete operation.

 Only users can view the audit trail for health items by using HealthVault Shell's history functionality. Applications do not have access to the audit trail of a health item.

Patient Connect

Several clinical applications use HealthVault to send information to consumers either a single time or continually through backend systems. CreateConnectPackage allows applications to create a one-time package for the user to receive in his HealthVault account, and DeleteConnectPackage allows applications to perform cleanup as necessary. On the other hand, CreateConnectRequest allows applications to establish a continual link with a patient's HealthVault record. Applications can get the details needed to make the link by using GetAuthorizedConnectRequests.

 HealthVault will delete the validated connect requests after a period of time. It is advised that applications calls GetAuthorizedConnectRequests daily or weekly to ensure that all validated connect requests are retrieved.

Asynchronous processing

HealthVault provides several mechanisms for an application to perform asynchronous processing. GetAuthorizedPeople gets information about the people that are authorized to use the application. This function paginates results using a `PersonID` cursor and provides a way to query authorizations created after a given point in time. Applications have found this function useful to send email updates and reminders to their subscribers. Similarly, GetUpdatedRecordsForApplication retrieves a list of records for an application with things that have been updated since a specified date.

HealthVault provides a powerful publish/subscribe mechanism. Applications can subscribe to events around create, read, update, and delete operations on HealthVault thing types. These events are registered with the platform using the `SubscribeToEvent` method. In addition to defining the subscribe event, the application registers a secure URI to which the HealthVault platform publishes events. The HealthVault eventing mechanism is documented in detail with appropriate examples at *http://msdn.microsoft.com/en-us/library/gg681193.aspx*.

The InstantPHR application from GetReal Consulting (*http://www.getrealconsulting.com/instantphr/*) is a good example of an application that uses HealthVault's asynchronous processing and eventing in particular to notify users of changes in their health records.

Messaging

Applications using HealthVault can send email messages to HealthVault users. The SendInsecureMessageFromApplication API allows the application to choose the sender address and specify its domain.

The HealthVault Messaging APIs are insecure. It would be better for an institution to set up the Direct email protocol and send secure email to the HealthVault user. HealthVault users get free Direct email addresses.

Terminology

Terminologies, also known as vocabularies, are a list of codes associated with well-known terms in a particular domain. HealthVault hosts numerous terminologies. Most of these are tagged as wc and are created by Microsoft. However, several third-party terminologies from the National Library of Medicine, USDA, HL7, and other institutions are also hosted.

You can use the PowerShell HealthVault plug-in to verify that Health-Vault hosts approximately 150 terminologies:

```
PS C:\> (Get-Vocabulary).Count
150
```

The terminologies can be accessed using the GetVocabulary API. Accessing the terminologies does not require user authentication; these are application-only APIs. Some terminologies hosted by HealthVault, such as RxNorm, are huge. RxNorm is a terminology that attempts to normalize all medication names and contains more than 200,000 entries. The SearchVocabulary API provides an XML interface as well as a JSON interface to search vocabularies. In fact, one can get an auto-completion text box for entering a medication by using SearchVocabulary on RxNorm. The HealthVault user interface provides auto-completion for medications, conditions, and other health item types using the SearchVocabulary API.

Application management

The SetApplicationSettings and GetApplicationSettings APIs provide a way for applications to store and retrieve their record-specific settings in HealthVault. Information such as theme selection by a particular user or order of authorized records can be stored in application settings. The multiple record management (MRA) functionality detailed later in this chapter can be implemented using these APIs.

HealthVault also allows a certain kind of application called a Master Application to create and manage other applications. Master Applications use the AddApplication and UpdateApplication functions to manage the "child" applications they create.

 There are very few Master Applications in the HealthVault ecosystem. The GoLive or publication bar for these applications is high. Once an application of this type is created, it cannot be deleted.

Service discovery

The GetServiceDefinition function provides access to all the details of HealthVault applications, including Methods, Schemas, and Configurations for the service. Using GetServiceDefinition, an application can programmatically discover HealthVault service information and keep it up to date.

 You can use the PowerShell HealthVault plug-in (Example 3-2) to explore GetServiceDefinition.

Example 3-2. Using GetServiceDefinition in HvPosh

```
PS C:\Windows\system32> Get-ServiceDefinition

HealthServiceUrl       : https://platform.healthvault-ppe.com/platform/wildcat.ashx
Version                : 1.9.2679.7415
HealthServiceShellInfo : Microsoft.Health.HealthServiceShellInfo
Assemblies             : {}
Methods                : {AddApplication, AllocatePackageId, AssociateAlternateId,
                         BeginPutBlob...}
IncludedSchemaUrls     : {https://platform.healthvault-ppe.com/platform/XSD/types.xsd,
                         https://platform.healthvault-ppe.com/platform/XSD/auth.xsd,
                         https://platform.healthvault-ppe.com/platform/XSD/application.xsd,
                         https://platform.healthvault-ppe.com/platform/XSD/vocab.xsd...}
ConfigurationValues    : {[allowedDocumentExtensions, .avi,.bluebutton,.bmp,.ccd,.ccr,.cda,
                         .doc,.docm,.docx,.eml,.gif,.jpg,.mp3,.one,.pdf,.png,.ppsm,.ppsx,
                         .ppt,.pptm,.pptx,.pub,.rpmsg,.rtf,.scp,.tif,.tiff,.txt,.vsd,.wav,
                         .wma,.wmv,.xls,.xlsb,.xlsm,.xlsx,.xltx,.xml,.xps],
                         [autoReconcilableTypes, 1e1ccbfc-a55d-4d91-8940-fa2fbf73c195,
                         9c48a2b8-952c-4f5a-935d-f3292326bf54], [blobHashBlockSizeBytes,
                         2097152], [blobHashDefaultAlgorithm, SHA256Block]...}
```

Open Query

Open Query is an insecure mechanism for running preconfigured queries invoked with an identifier on HealthVault data. For example, the following query:

https://platform.healthvault.com/platform/openquery.ashx?id=9C4C77CF-1DF0-4c41-BD3D-EC9232B5BC8A

invokes a saved request that corresponds to the specified identifier. Only queries associated with GetThings can be saved with SaveOpenQuery. The invocation of the open query doesn't require authentication and authorization, and the HealthVault team discourages its use and might remove it in future updates.

Read and Write API: Diving Deep

The most important HealthVault functions an application should become familiar with are GetThings and PutThings. In the following sections we will dive deeper in to each of these functions, discuss their treatment in the HealthVault .NET SDK, and see some examples. The code in this chapter can be a starting point for the more complex applications introduced in the rest of this book.

GetThings

The best way to understand GetThings API is to look at the XML that an application would send to HealthVault platform to request a set of things (Example 3-3).

Example 3-3. GetThings XML request

```
<wc-request:request xmlns:wc-request="urn:com.microsoft.wc.request">
  <auth>...</auth>
  <header>...</header>
  <info>
    <group name="GetWeights" max="10"> ❶
      <id>d8460ea8-50d4-4c30-ad92-49d1a1020b52</id>
      <filter>
        <type-id>d8460ea8-50d4-4c30-ad92-49d1a1020b52</type-id> ❷
        <thing-state>Active</thing-state> ❸
        <created-app-id>1F82D899-22E0-43F2-A645-59EDB6927645</created-app-id> ❹
        <xpath>/thing/data-xml/weight/value/kg[.>=60]</xpath> ❺
      </filter>
      <format>
        <section>core</section> ❻
        <xml /> ❼
      </format>
      <current-version-only>true</current-version-only> ❽
    </group>
  </info>
</wc-request:request>
```

Each GetThings request can have multiple queries called a group (Line ❶). Each group is identified by its name. The response from HealthVault combines the items returned by the group; group-name is used to index items returned for a particular query group. The group element can take one or more attributes to control the results. The attribute used in the previous example is max, which tells the HealthVault platform to return the top 10 items for this query.

Each query group can contain <filter> subelements to return particular items with a specific identification. Example 3-3 requests items with a specific type-id (Line ❷). The d84..52 identifier is associated with a particular instance of the weight type. Multiple IDs can be specified in each request. Other elements, such as client identifiers and thing keys, can also be used instead of an ID. The filter also restricts results to those that have an active thing-state (Line ❸) and were created using the Withings application (Line ❹). Items also can be filtered using XPath; on Line ❺ we are looking for weight items whose values are greater than 60 kg, maybe because we know that the scale was misconfigured during this time. To sum up, the query in Example 3-3 returns the core XML sections of the top 10 weight elements that were created by the Withings application and have values greater than 60 kg.

The format and quantity of information returned by the GetThings query can be controlled by format specifiers. Using the section tag, we can specify that we just want the core elements of the requested thing types (Line ❻). Other section tags could specify digital signatures, audit information, or effective permissions for the request. Using the xml tag (Line ❼), one can run an XSL transform on the thing types or choose from existing transforms available for the type. Our xml tag is empty, so no transform is run in the sample query. We will discuss MTT, STT, and other transforms in Chapter 4.

An application can request only the current versions of HealthVault thing types (Line ❽), although the platform does store older versions of the data.

To complete the discussion on the format of the GetThings request, note that I have collapsed the auth and header tags at the beginning of the code block. These elements specify the authorization information for the method and various other header elements, such as the method name, final-xsl, version, user, and application tokens.

Table 3-4 summarizes the querying ability of the GetThings method. To learn more, please refer to the methods schema documentation at *http://developer.healthvault.com/ pages/methods/methods.aspx* and associated HealthVault SDK reference at *http://msdn .microsoft.com/en-us/library/hh672196.aspx*.

Table 3-4. GetThings query parameters

Search Criteria	.NET SDK name	XML element	Name description
Group Attribute	Name	name	Identifies the group
	Max	max	Maximum number of things to be returned
	Max-Full	max-full	Maximum number of full things
Identifiers	ClientItemIds	client-thing-id	Client ID of the thing
	ItemIds	Id	Thing instance ID
	ItemKeys	key	Thing key
Filters	EffectiveDateMax	eff-date-max	Various thing filters
	EffectiveDateMin	eff-date-min	
	UpdatedDateMax	updated-date-max	
	UpdatedDateMin	updated-date-min	
	CreatedDateMax	created-date-max	
	CreatedDateMin	created-date-min	
	CreatedPerson	created-person-id	
	UpdatedPerson	updated-person-id	
	CreatedApplication	created-app-id	
	UpdatedApplication	updated-app-id	
	XPath	xpath	
	States	thing-state	
Formats	View	Section	Section to be retrieved (core, audits, effective permissions, digital signatures)
		Xml	Name of the transform to apply
		type-version-format	Version ID of the type format
		blob-payload-request	Sequence of blob-filters (BLOB names) and blob-format-spec (information, inline or streamed)
Versions	CurrentVersionOnly	current-version-only	

Now that we understand the paradigm through which one can access things from HealthVault using the GetThings methods, let's look at how we can utilize querying to display weight values in our application.

Our application currently fetches all the weight readings. However, we want to be able to explore the readings on a graph one week at a time. Example 3-4 shows how we can do it. As Line ❶ shows, we begin by creating a searcher object for the record we are working with, and then create a new filter for the weight type (Line ❷). Once we have the filter, we add properties to filter the value so that we get only those weight items that are dated for the previous week using EffectiveDateMin (Line ❸).

Once the query is constructed, we issue a GetThings request to HealthVault (Line ❹). Because we have only one group, we index for the results in the first set of matching results (GetMatchingItems()[0]).

Example 3-4. Using the EffectiveDateMin filter to get weekly data

```
protected void Btn_ShowWeeklyWeightReadings_Click(object sender, EventArgs e)
{
    HealthRecordSearcher searcher = PersonInfo.SelectedRecord.CreateSearcher(); ❶
    HealthRecordFilter filter = new HealthRecordFilter(Weight.TypeId); ❷
    filter.EffectiveDateMin = DateTime.Now.Subtract(new TimeSpan(7, 0, 0, 0)); ❸
    searcher.Filters.Add(filter);

    HealthRecordItemCollection items = searcher.GetMatchingItems()[0]; ❹

    TimeSeries t = new TimeSeries("Weight Graph"); ❺

    foreach (Weight item in items)
    {
        //Assuming all data is in one unit
        t.SeriesValue.Add(new TimeSeries.TimeSeriesValues(
            item.EffectiveDate, item.Value.DisplayValue.Value));
    }
    TimeplotView.Plots.Add(t); ❻
    TimeplotView.DataBind();
    TimeplotView.Visible = true;
}
```

After getting the matching items, we create a new TimeSeries (Line ❺) and add each item individually to the series. The *TimeSeries.ascx.cs* file contains an implementation of this class. You can choose to use your own implementation with any other graphing library. In this example, I'm using the Flot JavaScript graphing library (*http://code.goo gle.com/p/flot/*). TimeplotView (Line ❻) is an instance of a user control that has a Flot graphing object.

In the last three lines we add the constructed TimeSeries to the graphing object and make it visible on the screen. Figure 3-3 shows the results of running this query on the selected record.

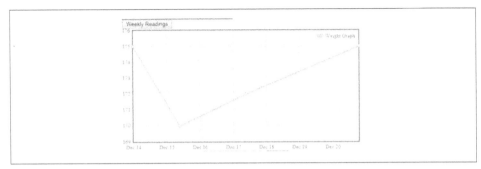

Figure 3-3. Filtering weight data for the week

PutThings

As with GetThings, we'll begin our coverage of the PutThings API by looking at the XML an application would send to HealthVault to create or update a set of things. Compared to GetThings, this is a simple request (Example 3-5).

Example 3-5. PutThings XML sample

```
<wc-request:request xmlns:wc-request="urn:com.microsoft.wc.request">
  <auth>
    <hmac-data algName="HMACSHA1">IB7cdWXFNKE+xhrvE5poT5uluEE=</hmac-data>
  </auth>
  <header>...</header>
  <info>
    <thing> ❶
      <type-id>0a5f9a43-dc88-4e9f-890f-1f9159b76e7b</type-id> ❷
      <thing-state>Active</thing-state>
      <data-xml>...</data-xml> ❸
    </thing>
  </info>
</wc-request:request>
```

Each PutThings request can add instances of a thing (Line ❶). Each thing has a type-id (Line ❷) that identifies what kind of data item it is. In Example 3-5, the thing is of type Weight. Because we are adding a weight thing, the data-xml (Line ❸) part of this request needs to adhere to the schema for this particular type. In Chapter 4, we will discuss the thing-type schema. The important aspect of using this schema is to make sure to use a unique thing-id. In case of an update, the thing-id is the instance of weight you want to update. Additionally, the thing-version-id element should be the version ID of the element that is currently in the HealthVault. HealthVault offers optimistic concurrency, which means that if an application tries to update an old thing that has already been updated by some other application, its version ID will have changed and the new put won't succeed. The thing-version-id is critical to make sure one update does not override another.

Let's modify our application to add a new `Weight` element to HealthVault. On the *Default.aspx* page, we construct a text box to enter weight in pounds and associate a "save" button with it, with the action as `Btn_SubmitWeight_Click`.

Example 3-6 illustrates how we will go about saving a new element to HealthVault. Notice the HealthVault-specific `DateTime` field (`HealthServiceDateTime`) on Line ❶ and a way to differentiate the actual `WeightValue` from `DisplayValue` on Lines ❷–❸. HealthVault enables health items to have a flexible date and time. It also stores measurements in a canonical format and allows users to see them in the format in which they entered the data.

In the case of `Weight`, it is stored canonically in kilograms, but we assume the user prefers to enter and display the weight in pounds. So, on Line ❸ we multiply the value entered by the user by 1.6. The `DisplayValue` of the weight is in pounds (`lbs`), which the applications working with this type can use to show the value to the user.

Example 3-6. PutThings example

```
protected void Btn_SubmitWeight_Click(object sender, EventArgs e)
{
    double weight = double.Parse(Txt_Weight.Text);
    Weight w = new Weight(
            new HealthServiceDateTime(DateTime.Now), ❶
            new WeightValue( ❷
                weight * 1.6, new DisplayValue(weight, "lbs", "lbs"))); ❸

    PersonInfo.SelectedRecord.NewItem(w);
}
```

Having a well-formed weight health item, we can send it to HealthVault by calling the `NewItem` method in the HealthVault .NET SDK. Under the hood, the `NewItem` call issues a PutThings request to the HealthVault platform. The HealthVault SDK also has an `UpdateItem` method, which saves changes to an existing item using the `PutThings` method.

To update an existing item, one essentially does the same thing as shown, except you use the `UpdateItem` SDK method instead of `NewItem`.

 The code in Java shown in Example 3-7 is equivalent to the .NET in Example 3-6. The OnlineRequestTemplate is generated using the library's SimpleRequestTemplate, and it sets an appropriate User-AuthToken and PersonId on the request.

Example 3-7. Reading weight using the Java SDK

```java
public void PutThing() throws Exception
    {
        long weightValueInKg = 80;

        DisplayValue dv = new DisplayValue();
        dv.setUnits("lb");
        dv.setUnitsCode("lb");
        dv.setValue(weightValueInKg/2.2);

        WeightValue wv = new WeightValue();
        wv.setKg(weightValueInKg);
        wv.setDisplay(dv);

        Weight weight = new Weight();
        weight.setValue(wv);
        weight.setWhen(DateTime.fromCalendar(Calendar.getInstance()));

        Thing thing = new Thing();
        thing.setData(weight);

        SimpleRequestTemplate requestTemplate = new SimpleRequestTemplate(
                ConnectionFactory.getConnection());
        requestTemplate.setPersonId("75ac2c6c-c90e-4f7e-b74d-bb7e81787beb");
        requestTemplate.setRecordId("8c390004-3d41-4f5c-8f24-4841651579d6");

        PutThingsRequest request = new PutThingsRequest();
        request.getThing().add(thing);

        PutThingsResponse response =
(PutThingsResponse)requestTemplate.makeRequest(request);
    }
```

Record Management: Diving Deep

Single-record application (SRA)

For an application working with a single record, HealthVault provides a simple mechanism to switch to another record using a switch record hyperlink. In order for an application to switch to a different record, the application needs to tell the HealthVault Shell to allow the user to switch the record and have a preconfigured receiving end point for the HealthVault Shell to send the user back to a notification to change the selected record, termed a SELECTEDRECORD. The application redirects the user with a hyperlink URL like the one shown in the following example. The *AUTH* target implies an authentication request, the *appid* implies the identifier associated with the calling application, and the *forceappauth* string makes sure that the user is able to change the record.

https://account.healthvault-ppe.com/redirect.aspx?target=AUTH&targetqs=appid %3D82d47a5a-d435-4246-895a-746c475090d3%26forceappauth%3Dtrue

Using the HealthVault .NET Web SDK, this can be done with following line of code. The last variable enables applications to pass any optional parameters that need to pass through the URL redirection:

```
this.RedirectToShellUrl("AUTH", "appid=" + this.ApplicationId.ToString() +
"&forceappauth=true", "passthroughParam=optional");
```

As a simple example, Figure 3-4 shows how one can associate the Switch Account functionality to an existing HealthVault application. Enabling this functionality involves two steps. First is to create an appropriate URL to send the user to HealthVault; Example 3-8 shows the associated code. The second step in this process is to create a receiving URL so that HealthVault can send the user back to your application. Example 3-9 shows the associated code required to configure a SelectedRecordChanged endpoint page in the HealthVault SDK's *web.config* file. These two steps are relatively simple and can be accomplished with any programming language. "HealthVault Shell Interface" on page 28 explains the HealthVault shell interface, and "HealthVault SDK and Open Source Libraries" on page 43 lists the available libraries.

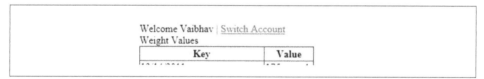

Figure 3-4. Adding the ability to switch accounts

In Example 3-8, notice that in Line ❶, we are using the RedirectToShellUrl HealthVault SDK functionality to enable creating the appropriate redirection URL for HealthVault.

Example 3-8. Adding a redirect URL in Default.aspx.cs

```
protected void Lnk_SwitchAccount_Click(object sender, EventArgs e)
{
    this.RedirectToShellUrl("AUTH", "appid=" + this.ApplicationId.ToString() + ❶
        "&forceappauth=true", "passthroughParam=optional");
}
```

In Example 3-9, we are creating a key in the *web.config* file to associate a receiving end point for the selected "record changed" action. In the next section, we explain the HealthVault shell interface in detail.

Example 3-9. Handling a SelectRecordChanged target in web.config

```
<!-- Handling selected record changed -->
<add key="WCPage_ActionSelectedRecordChanged" value="default.aspx"/>
```

Multiple-record application (MRA)

The Mayo Clinic Health Manager works with all the records associated with the account and functions as a multiple-record application (MRA). As illustrated in Figure 3-5, I can switch from my record to my mom's record seamlessly within the Mayo Clinic application. This flexibility can be achieved in an application by including `IsMRA=true` while communicating with HealthVault Shell's Authentication (AUTH) mechanism, as detailed in "HealthVault Shell Interface" on page 28. Using this capability, the application can then authenticate multiple records at the same time and make requests to access health information for each one of them. For the application to remember the previous active record before switching to any associated record, it should store the current record identifier in the application settings associated with the person before making the switch.

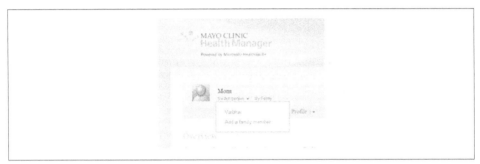

Figure 3-5. An application working with multiple records

HealthVault SDK and Open Source Libraries

The HealthVault team offers a .NET SDK available at *http://www.msdn.com/health vault*. Additionally, a number of open source libraries offer higher-level abstractions for interacting with the HealthVault platform. This section outlines the level of abstractions available in each of these libraries.

HealthVault .NET SDK

The HealthVault .NET SDK is the official software development kit available from Microsoft for working with the HealthVault platform. The HealthVault team maintains this SDK and provides interfaces for all HealthVault interfaces.

This SDK does not support the HealthVault Client APIs for mobile phones, but it does support the HealthVault Client APIs for Windows Applications. The Shell Redirect Interface is supported, but not all capabilities are supported. Notably, this is the only SDK that supports signing health items and streaming large files to HealthVault. HealthVault uses Azure, Microsoft's cloud storage service, to store these large files.

Throughout this book, we will be looking at code that uses this SDK, and refer to it as the HealthVault .NET SDK. Officially each major release of this SDK is supported for two years, and the SDK is currently compatible with .NET framework version 2.0.

The source code of this SDK is available for reference, but the license terms don't allow modifications to the SDK.

HealthVault Open Source Java SDK

This is the second most popular SDK for the HealthVault platform. The HealthVault open source Java SDK is available under a very permissive open source license at *http: //healthvaultjavalib.codeplex.com*. This SDK was developed by members of the Health-Vault team and provides interfaces for most HealthVault interfaces. The source code of the SDK is available under the Microsoft Public License, and modifications and redistribution of this code are permitted for commercial and noncommercial purposes.

Notably, this SDK supports the HealthVault Client APIs for Android mobile phones, and it provides a complete abstraction layer for Shell redirect interfaces. But it does not support Patient Connect, asynchronous processes, signing of health items, or streaming large files to HealthVault. However, there are samples or documentation available for signing and streaming.

Additionally, the SDK provides an object wrapper for thing types using code generation tools. If these classes don't meet your needs, you can use the method schemas and create suitable wrappers.

This SDK is fully available for JDK 1.6; however, raw authentication is supported for JDK 1.4. The SDK is community supported, and patches for bug fixes or missing functionality are welcomed.

Certificate Management

For the .NET SDK and Windows platform, the HealthVault SDK offers the Application Manager tool to make it easy to work with public and private keys for your application. In the case of Java, the best way to handle certificates for the application is to create one using the keytool from the Java SDK.

The following **keytool** command creates a public and private key pair for your application in the Java **keystore**:

```
keytool -genkeypair -keyalg RSA -keysize 2048 -keystore keystore -alias
java-wildcat -validity 9999
```

Note that the algorithm used is RSA and the **keysize** is 2 kilobytes; it's recommend to have the **keysize** as large as your installation supports. The generated key pair is valid for 9,999 days, and you can choose to configure it. The name of the key pair is **java-wildcat**, which needs to be added to the *hv-application.properties* file in the Java SDK.

The HealthVault platform needs to have the certificate associated with the public key of your application. The keytool can also be used to export this certificate. The following is a sample command to do this:

```
keytool -export -alias java-wildcat -keystore keystore > my-pub.cer
```

Here `java-wildcat` is the name of the application's key pair and it's exported as *my-pub.cer*.

HealthVault Open Source iOS Mobile Library

The HealthVault team provides an open source and community-supported library for the iOS platform available at *https://github.com/microsoft-hsg/HealthVault-Mobile-iOS-Library*. This library provides basic functionality to authenticate mobile clients. It doesn't provide support for any additional HealthVault features.

Applications such as iTriage (*http://www.itriagehealth.com/*) have used this library to create HealthVault iOS applications.

This library is available under the Apache 2.0 open source license, and modifications and redistribution of this code are permitted for commercial and noncommercials purposes.

HealthVault Open Source Windows Phone Library

Like the iOS library, the Windows Phone library at *http://healthvaultwp7.codeplex.com/* provides an authentication abstraction for Windows Phone mobile clients. Applications such LiveScape (*http://livescape.mobi/*) have used this library to create HealthVault-enabled Windows Phone applications.

This library is available under the Apache 2.0 open source license, and modifications and redistribution of this code are permitted for commercial and noncommercials purposes.

In Chapter 5, we will walk through a detailed application that shows how to work with HealthVault mobile interfaces.

HealthVault Open Source Python, PHP, and Ruby Library

The HealthVault team has helped create Python, PHP, and Ruby libraries. These libraries are primarily driven by partners and provide the basic authentication layer for working with the HealthVault service. Applications such as TrailX (Python), Teladoc (PHP), and podfitness (Ruby) have used these libraries to create successful HealthVault applications.

These libraries are available under the Apache 2.0 open source license, and modifications and redistribution of this code are permitted for commercial and noncommercial purposes.

Table 3-5 summarizes the functionality available in various HealthVault libraries.

Table 3-5. HealthVault SDK and open source libraries

SDK library	Distribution	Supported platform	Features available	License and support
HealthVault .NET	MSDN	Windows XP, Vista, 7 (.NET 2.0)	All HealthVault features	Microsoft Reciprocal License (MS-RL)
				Microsoft supported
Java	Codeplex	JDK 1.6	Authentication, method wrappers, thing-type wrappers	Microsoft Public License (MS-PL)
		JDK 1.4 (limited)		Community support
Java	Codeplex	Android (1.6+)	Authentication, thing-type wrappers	MS-PL
				Community support
iOS	GitHub	iOS 4.0+	Mobile authentication	Apache 2.0
				Community Support
Windows Phone	Codeplex	Windows Phone 7+	Mobile authentication	Apache 2.0
				Community support
Python	Google Code	Python 2.7	Authentication (basic)	Apache 2.0
				Community support
PHP	SourceForge	PHP	Authentication (basic)	Apache 2.0
				Community support
Ruby	RubyForge	Ruby	Authentication (basic)	Apache 2.0
				Community support

Interfacing with HealthVault

We touched on the HealthVault APIs and interface; these interfaces are usually combined in multiple ways to create integration architectures with HealthVault. This section discusses high-level options for integrating applications and devices with Health-Vault. This discussion should be useful for understanding different architectural patterns available for interfacing devices and applications with HealthVault.

Device Connectivity

As of this writing, more than 80 types of devices connect with HealthVault. These devices range from pedometers and weighing scales to blood pressure meters and pulse oximeters. Figure 3-6 shows the various interfaces available for a device to connect with HealthVault.

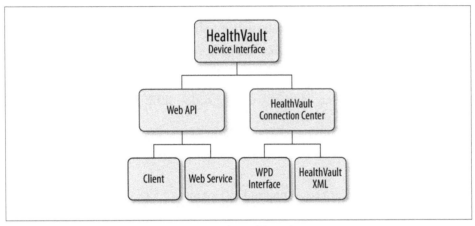

Figure 3-6. Interfaces for device integration with HealthVault

Currently, a large number of devices interface with HealthVault through HealthVault's Windows client utility, called HealthVault Connection Center. HealthVault Connection Center enables device integration using the Windows Portable Devices (WPD) standard.

If a device already has a Windows device driver, the appropriate data can be communicated to HealthVault using the WPD standard. The HealthVault team has a device development kit (DDK) that can be used for this integration, but its use lies outside the scope of this book.

When there are no WPD-supported elements for a device, it can still integrate with HealthVault through the HealthVault Connection Center by sending and receiving HealthVault XML directly. Chapter 4 describes the HealthVault's XML data types. This approach is referred to as HealthVault XML in Figure 3-6. The HealthVault DDK has an example of how to go about configuring such an interface.

In addition to interfacing devices through the HealthVault Connection Center, device manufacturers can write their own client application to enable data to upload to HealthVault using the HealthVault Client SDKs. ECG Glove, which is available at *http://ineedmd.com/*, is a good example of a device that sends information to HealthVault using this interface.

Devices such as Fitbit and Withings actually take integration a step further and interface with HealthVault directly through the cloud using HealthVault APIs.

Continua

Continua Health Alliance is a nonprofit, open industry organization of health care and technology companies joining together to improve the quality of personal connected health care. With more than 230 member companies around the world, it is the leading consortium for personal health care devices. HealthVault has announced that support for Continua drivers will be available in the future. When this happens, devices will be able to play well in the HealthVault and Continua ecosystem, either by using the HealthVault Web API or by converting data into IEEE 11073 formats.

Continua is not a standards body, but has identified a set of standards that together enable a personal connected health care ecosystem. At its heart is the IEEE 11073 Personal Health Data Standard, which dictates various data standard profiles for devices ranging from blood pressure cuffs to weighing scales. IEEE 11073 is a data standard and is independent of transport.

On the transport layer, Continua supports USB personal Health Class devices, Bluetooth health care device profiles, and other transports as they become compliant in the future.

Figure 3-7 shows the interfaces supported by Continua.

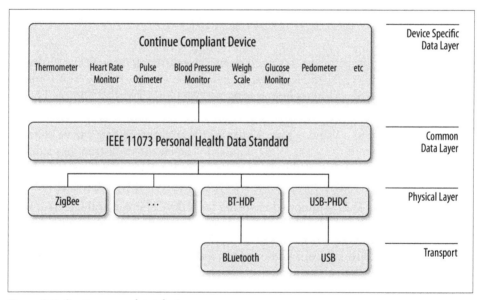

Figure 3-7. Continua-complaint devices

Application Connectivity

As of this writing, there are more than 300 HealthVault applications are live in the United States. HealthVault applications work with the HealthVault personal health data store by using various APIs over the HTTP protocol, as we have seen with Put-Things and GetThings. Figure 3-8 depicts various ways in which applications have interfaced with HealthVault, depending on their use case.

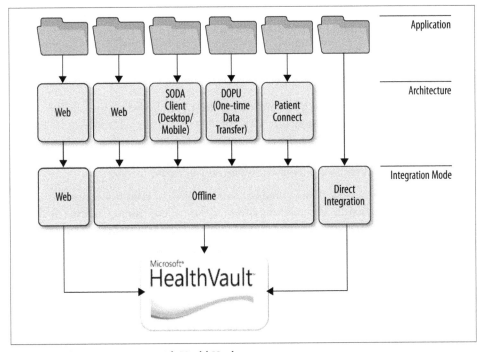

Figure 3-8. Connectivity types with HealthVault

The following discussion goes into detail about various modes of connecting with HealthVault, which depend on the applications' needs as they pertain to the underlying platform, user consent, authentication, and user interface.

Online HealthVault application

In addition to data storage, native HealthVault applications can use HealthVault for user authentication and authorization. Any data accessed using this mode requires the user's explicit permission each time the application interacts with HealthVault.

Mayo Clinic Health Manager, *https://healthmanager.mayoclinic.com/*, is a native HealthVault application.

Offline HealthVault application

Applications can choose to simply store and access data from HealthVault without using HealthVault as a primary authentication and authorization entity.

FitBit (*http://www.fitbit.com/*) is a good example of an offline application. It links a FitBit account with a HealthVault user record and account, and then interacts with the health items therein.

Drop Off Pick Up. Drop Off Pick Up (DOPU) is analogous to sending a secured fax to a HealthVault user. The data flow in this architecture is one-way. The application drops the data into HealthVault, and the user picks it up.

If a consumer happens to visit a health care institution and does not intend to have an ongoing relationship with the care entity, DOPU provides an effective mechanism for the institution to provide documents.

Patient Connect. Some entities don't intend to maintain a public-facing website but would like to have an ongoing relationship with their users through HealthVault. Patient Connect provides an ideal mechanism for such institutions. Via this mechanism, the user authorizes an application to read or write data to her HealthVault record through a user interface on HealthVault.com (*http://healthvault.com*).

Clinical systems such as electronic medical records (EMRs) commonly use this model to connect to HealthVault, which is why this model is called Patient Connect. It should be noted, however, that this model is not limited to clinical systems and can be used by any backend system.

Client Connectivity. Client Connectivity, referred to as Software on Device Authentication (SODA), enables applications to run on client platforms like desktop or mobile device, outside of the web browser. Every time a user installs a SODA application, the user must authorize that installation of the application to access his HealthVault record. For instance, if the user is running the same application on both his laptop and desktop, he will need to authorize both installations to access his HealthVault record.

A number of mobile health applications (such as iTriage, LiveScape, and Weight4Me) use this architecture. In Chapter 5 we will develop a mobile application and do a detailed walkthrough of the APIs available to use this type of interface.

Direct integration

The Direct project, formerly known as NHIN Direct, is collaboration between the public and private sector to develop a simple, secure, and standards-based method to send encrypted health information directly to known, trusted recipients over the Internet. This project aims at replacing the fax machine in health care. Providers are able to send documents to each other securely.

Direct integration is the easiest kind of integration with HealthVault, and trusted applications can actually send and receive documents to and from HealthVault using a Direct-enabled email address. HealthVault users get an email address in the format *<handle>@direct.healthvault.com*. As part of its Direct implementation, HealthVault automatically adds any recognized attachments (for example, CCDs or CCRs) to the user's record.

Google Health was able to interface with HealthVault using the Direct integration. For HealthVault to accept emails from a new direct domain, the application needs to register the public key with HealthVault. If the application sends email to *newuser@direct.healthvault.com* with the user's email address in the subject line, HealthVault stores the email in a password-encrypted package and sends an email to the user to associate the dropped-off information to their record. The user can also sign into her HealthVault record and read the message in the HealthVault Message Center.

Application Provisioning and master applications

Application Provisioning refers to providing an application in HealthVault's production environment, which the HeathVault team does for all of the connectivity models discussed so far. However, in special cases it provides the ability for applications known as "master" applications to provision individual HealthVault "child" applications.

Frequently, solution providers develop HealthVault integration for common scenarios such as uploading lab information or sending clinical care record information from a facility's EMR system. These solutions are deployed separately for each institution. The HealthVault team delegates the responsibility for creating these individual application instances to the solution provider through the Master Application mechanism.

Thus, for instance, if we wanted to deploy an individual instance of a Weight Tracker application per institution, we would use the AddApplication API available from the HealthVault Platform. "Further Resources" on page 99 has links to examples and resources about how to create a child application.

CHAPTER 4

Using the HealthVault Data Ecosystem for Self-Tracking

"Data is a precious thing and will last longer than the systems themselves."

—Tim Bernes-Lee

The Quantified Self (*http://quantifiedself.com/about/*) community enables self-knowledge through self-tracking. Self-tracking, when powered by appropriate data analysis, has been proven to trigger behavioral change. The act of self-tracking creates awareness and feedback. The hunger for, and success of, self-knowledge is evident from the growing number of self-quantifiers (currently 6,000+ in 41 cities and 14 countries).

Self-knowledge is possible only with a substantial collection of data about oneself. HealthVault provides more than 80 granular data types that enable tracking data regarding everything from daily exercise to genome sequences. In this chapter, we will build upon the understanding of the HealthVault API covered in Chapter 3 and extend it to develop a data-intensive self-quantifying application. Through the Quantified Self application, we will gain an understanding of HealthVault data types and application development.

A Self-Experimentation Application

In Chapter 1 we analyzed weight data, and in Chapter 2 we worked with sleep information and correlated it with exercise. HealthVault offers a data type for tracking emotional state and daily dietary intake as well. Let's consider building a simple Quantified Self utility that helps a user keep track of his emotional state, daily dietary intake, weight, sleep, and exercise. Tracking these types of data and their relation to each other would allow our user to form and prove interesting hypotheses such as: "I'm happier if I sleep well, and I sleep well if I drink less alcohol and exercise sufficiently."

Self-tracking fosters awareness and a feedback loop; numerous participants in the Quantified Self movement have attributed improvement to insights generated by the data and the act of data collection. Our Quantified Self application will aim to emulate this pattern. Figure 4-1 summarizes the data pattern we wish to capture.

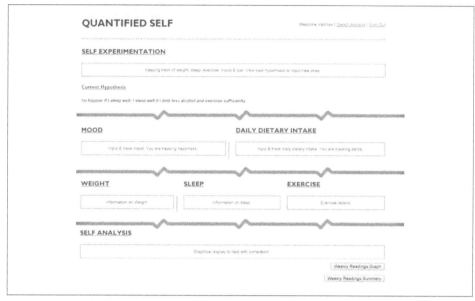

Figure 4-1. Data dashboard for Quantified Self application

Setting Up a New HealthVault Application

Let's start by making a Quantified Self application with a unique application identifier. In this chapter we will use the HealthVault .NET SDK in order to focus on understanding the HealthVault data types. However, as "HealthVault SDK and Open Source Libraries" on page 43 outlines, you can use other languages and HealthVault libraries as well.

The first step in creating the application is to download and install the HealthVault SDK from MSDN (*http://msdn.microsoft.com/en-us/healthvault*). After installing the SDK, you will notice a utility called Application Manager. From the Windows Start button, this utility can be accessed through All Programs→Microsoft Health-Vault→SDK→HealthVault Application Manager.

Once you open the Application Manager, you will notice the Create New Application button, which you should use now to create a new application. As Figure 4-2 shows, the new application creation process asks you for an application name and other details, and creates a Visual Studio solution with the application starting point.

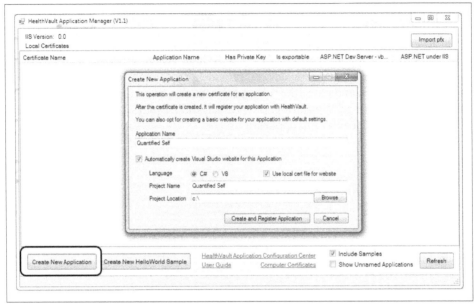

Figure 4-2. Using Application Manager to create a new HealthVault application

The second step in the process is to register your application. Application Manager automatically opens a new browser window that signs you into the HealthVault Application Configuration utility (*https://config.healthvault.com*) and creates the appropriate application in the HealthVault Development environment. The development environment is frequently referred to as PPE, which stands for preproduction environment. In the next chapter we will learn how the Application Configuration Center can be used to create a development application without using the Application Manager.

On the dashboard of the HealthVault Application Configuration Center, you will see the application you just created, as depicted in Figure 4-3.

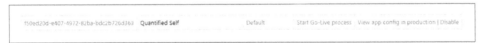

Figure 4-3. HealthVault Application Configuration Center showing the application that was created

Adding Data Types

HealthVault offers more than 80 granular items to which a user can authorize access. They fall into categories such as fitness, condition, medications, health history, measurements, personal profile, files, and custom data. A developer can obtain access for particular health data items by configuring an application's authorization rule set. For our application, we need access to weight, sleep, and exercise data, which come directly from various devices. We also want the user to be able to track emotional state and daily dietary intake, which is information that she will enter manually.

To start the necessary configuration, click on the application ID in the HealthVault Application Configuration Center. Figure 4-4 illustrates the view of our Quantified Self application after clicking on the "Online rules" tab. In this menu, select the appropriate data types for the application (weight measurement, sleep, exercise, etc.), select all permissions (read, write, update, delete), provide a reason why the application needs access to these types, and name the rule. A rule can also be configured as optional and can have display settings. Why String, Is Optional, and Display Flags items are currently not active for most HealthVault applications.

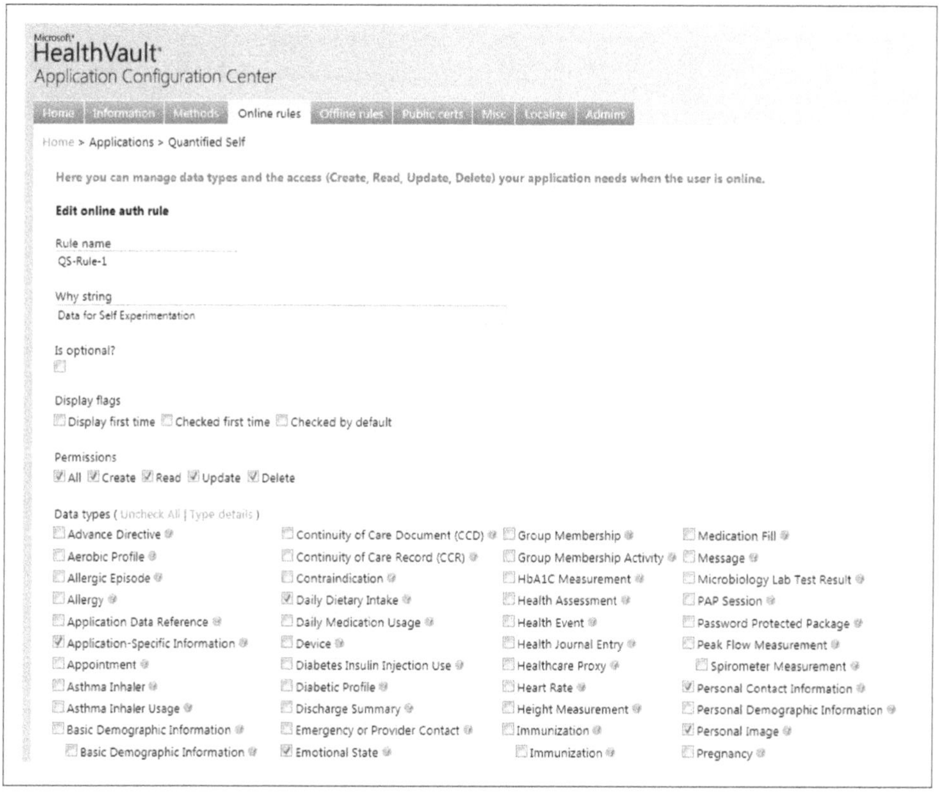

Figure 4-4. Configuring online rules for an application

We are using HealthVault as the user authentication provider for our application, so we choose to operate in the online mode and create an authorization rule for such access. If we wanted our application to work through a backend system provided by one of the other types of architecture discussed in Chapter 3, we would configure the offline rules for access to appropriate data types.

We are finished selecting the appropriate data types for our application, and can now try accessing them through the application.

Accessing the Data Types

The application manager utility creates a template application. Figure 4-5 shows the initial solution created by this utility.

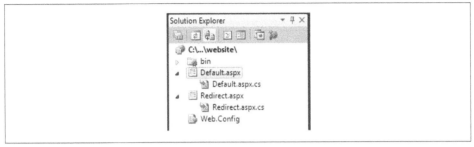

Figure 4-5. Solution created by the application manager

The solution makes sure that your application is configured properly with an appropriate application ID, points it to the appropriate HealthVault platform and shell development environments, and configures the application's redirect URL; all of these configurations live in the *Web.Config* file. The *Default.aspx* page is derived from the *HealthServicePage* and handles authorization with the HealthVault Platform, whereas the *Redirect.aspx* page is derived from the *HealthServiceActionPage* and handles authentication and interaction with HealthVault Shell. The *bin* folder contains Health-Vault SDK libraries: *Microsoft.Health.dll*, which encapsulates the core HealthVault functionality; *Microsoft.Health.Web.dll*, which broadly encapsulates browser interaction; and *Microsoft.Health.Itemtypes*, which encapsulates an object model for all HealthVault data types.

The main solution doesn't add a master page. In order to make it easy to extend functionality, we create a MasterPage named *QuantifiedSelf.master*, create a fresh *Default.aspx* page after deleting the old one, and ensure this page is derived from *HealthServicePage*.

As discussed in Chapter 3, we can use the HealthVault GetThings API to access health items in a user's health record. The code shown in Example 4-1 accesses `Emotion`, `DietaryDailyIntake`, `Weight`, `Sleep`, and `Exercise` from HealthVault. As shown in the two lines at ❶, we make sure to fetch these elements for the last seven days only.

Example 4-1. GetThings call to access multiple things

```
protected void Page_Load(object sender, EventArgs e)
{
    Lbl_UserName.Text = this.PersonInfo.SelectedRecord.DisplayName;

    HealthRecordSearcher searcher = PersonInfo.SelectedRecord.CreateSearcher();
    HealthRecordFilter filter = new HealthRecordFilter(
        ApplicationSpecific.TypeId,
        Emotion.TypeId,
```

```
DietaryDailyIntake.TypeId,
Weight.TypeId,
SleepJournalAM.TypeId,
Exercise.TypeId);

filter.EffectiveDateMin = DateTime.Now.Subtract(new TimeSpan(7, 0, 0, 0)); ❶
searcher.Filters.Add(filter);

HealthRecordItemCollection items = searcher.GetMatchingItems()[0];
```

Before we display these types, let's dig deeper to understand a HealthVault data type.

Understanding HealthVault Data Types

A comprehensive list of all HealthVault data types is available from the HealthVault developer center at *http://developer.healthvault.com/types/types.aspx*. Each type has properties that determine to a great extent how items are created and used. To understand a type better, let's take a deeper look at the example of the Weight Measurement type.

Type Properties

Figure 4-6 shows the properties of the Weight Measurement data type that are common to every data type from the HealthVault developer center (*http://developer.healthvault .com/types/type.aspx?id=3d34d87e-7fc1-4153-800f-f56592cb0d17*). Each HealthVault type has a unique identifier; this id is used by the HealthVault APIs to identify the type. In the case of Weight, it is 3d34d87e-7fc1-4153-800f-f56592cb0d17. A type sets the uncreateable property to true if no application can create such a type in a user's HealthVault record; a good example of this is the Basic type. The immutable property is true if no application can modify or update an instance of that type in the user's HealthVault record; a good example of this is the CCR type. The property singleton is true if only one instance of that type can exist in a user's HealthVault record; a good example of this is the Basic Demographic type.

Type transforms

Additionally, the list of transforms is a property associated with the type. Transforms are built-in XSLT transformations available for a particular thing type. These transforms let you convert the XML associated with a particular type to various formats, such as HTML, to a representation compatible with various popular health care standards, or to an older or newer version of the same type.

Form, STT, and MTT transforms. Common among all the types are the form, stt, and mtt transforms. form provides an HTML table representation of an instance of the entire thing. stt, which stands for "single type transform," provides a row- based representation of the type so that it can be viewed as a list of instances of the same type. mtt, or

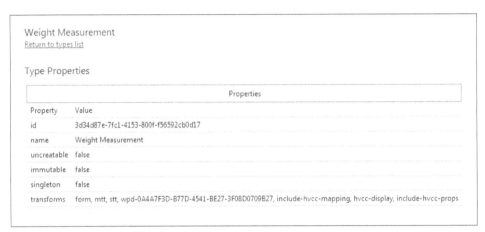

Figure 4-6. Properties of the Weight Measurement type

"multiple type transform," provides a row-based representation of the type so that it can be combined and viewed with multiple HealthVault types. Each row in `mtt` has a summary attribute representing the details of the type. The main difference between `stt` and `mtt` is that `stt` has an XML attribute for each meaningful data element of the type, whereas `mtt` summarizes all the meaningful data elements in one string in the `summary` attribute.

One can use the HealthVault PowerShell plug-in to view each source of the transforms. Example 4-2 shows how to save the `form` transform for the Weight thing type.

Example 4-2. Saving the form XSLT transformation for Weight thing types to a file

```
PS \> (Get-ThingType 3d34d87e-7fc1-4153-800f-f56592cb0d17).TransformSource["form"] |
out-file Weight.xsl
```

The columns on the type definition page in the HealthVault Type Explorer define the column header, .NET data type, and width for each column. It's handy to view this information about the type in a data grid.

Example 4-3 shows the multitype table transformation XML returned by the Health-Vault platform for the Weight type. We can see the columns ranging from `wc-id` (type identification) to `summary` (summary information of the type).

Example 4-3. Weight mtt XML for the Weight type

```
<data-xml transform="mtt">
  <row wc-id="34655fb4-a6c8-4d47-85f1-dbc6e09b952a"
    wc-version="0f57073a-0795-4867-9c9f-bcb99d2fa681" wc-note="" wc-tags=""
    wc-date="2011-12-23 11:17:47" wc-type="Weight Measurement"
    wc-typeid="3d34d87e-7fc1-4153-800f-f56592cb0d17" wc-source="" wc-brands=""
    wc-issigned="false" wc-flags="" wc-ispersonal="false" wc-isdownversioned="false"
    wc-isupversioned="false" wc-relatedthings="" wc-state="Active" summary="173 lbs" />
</data-xml>
```

In our Quantified Self application, we can use the mtt transform to easily display multiple types in the same table for self-analysis. In Example 4-4, Lines ❶–❸ construct and fetch our query from HealthVault; note that in Line ❷ we ask the HealthVault platform to apply the mtt transform on the returned items. In Line ❹, we select the row for each data-xml mtt transform. We then display the wc-date, wc-type, and summary columns (Lines ❺–❻). Different applications can choose to show different columns. Individual type columns, such as weight for Weight, are available in single type transform (stt), whereas a summary column summarizes this information in mtt. The HealthDataItem Grid control is also available from the HealthVault .NET SDK to show this information automatically.

Example 4-4. Viewing multiple HealthVault types in a data grid

```
protected void Btn_ShowWeeklyReadingsTextSummary_Click
    (object sender, System.EventArgs e)
{
    HealthRecordSearcher searcher = PersonInfo.SelectedRecord.CreateSearcher(); ❶
    HealthRecordFilter filter = new HealthRecordFilter(
        Emotion.TypeId,
        DietaryDailyIntake.TypeId,
        Weight.TypeId,
        SleepJournalAM.TypeId,
        Exercise.TypeId);

    filter.EffectiveDateMin = DateTime.Now.Subtract(new TimeSpan(7, 0, 0, 0));
    searcher.Filters.Add(filter);
    filter.View.TransformsToApply.Add("mtt"); ❷

    HealthRecordItemCollection items = searcher.GetMatchingItems()[0]; ❸

    DataTable dataTable = new DataTable();
    dataTable.Columns.Add(new DataColumn("Date", typeof(string)));
    dataTable.Columns.Add(new DataColumn("Type", typeof(string)));
    dataTable.Columns.Add(new DataColumn("Summary", typeof(string)));
    foreach (HealthRecordItem item in items)
    {
        XmlNode mttDocument = item.TransformedXmlData["mtt"] ❹
            .SelectSingleNode("data-xml/row");
        DataRow row = dataTable.NewRow();
        row["Date"] = mttDocument.Attributes["wc-date"].Value; ❺
        row["Type"] = mttDocument.Attributes["wc-type"].Value;
        row["Summary"] = mttDocument.Attributes["summary"].Value;
        dataTable.Rows.Add(row); ❻
    }

    Grid_ReadingsTextSummary.DataSource = dataTable;
    Grid_ReadingsTextSummary.DataBind();
    Grid_ReadingsTextSummary.Visible = true;
}
```

Once we have the data grid configured, we can view the summary of all types in the same column structure. Figure 4-7 shows how this information is displayed in our Quantified Self application.

Summary

Weekly Readings Summary

Date	Type	Summary
2012-03-11 21:00:27	Exercise	Walked 10,000 steps
2012-03-11 20:56:36	Weight Measurement	173 lbs
2012-03-11	Daily Dietary Intake	1000 kCal, carbs:500 g
2012-03-09	Weight Measurement	170 pounds
2012-03-08	Weight Measurement	171 pounds

Figure 4-7. Quantified Self application showing multiple types in a data grid

The CCR HealthVault type (1e1ccbfc-a55d-4d91-8940-fa2fbf73c195) has a `tohv` transform that converts the data in that type to individual HealthVault elements.

In addition to the use of transforms to convert types to different representations, the HealthVault method schema provides a `<final-xsl>` element in each method header. `final-xsl` converts the data returned by the method call to built-in transforms, such as converting to CCR (`toccr`), CCD (`toccd`), CSV (`tocsv`), or RSS (`torss`). `final-xsl` also allows the caller to specify a custom-built XSLT transform that the HealthVault platform runs on the output before sending it to the requester.

The `final-xsl` element is specified between the `<country>` and `<msg-time>` elements in the header of a method. In the HealthVault .NET SDK, one can call this functionality by using the `GetTransformedItems` method. In the Java .NET Open Source library, this functionality can be used through a call to `request.setFinalXsl("transform name or transform source")`.

Versioning transforms. HealthVault data types can have multiple versions. As the HealthVault ecosystem matures, existing types need to be updated or modified to match new use cases. Medications, Basic Demographic Information, and Family History are good examples of types that have multiple versions. You will notice that the older Medication datatype (which is available at *http://developer.healthvault.com/pages/types/type.aspx?id=5c5f1223-f63c-4464-870c-3e36ba471def*) has an up-version transform, and the newer Medication datatype (*http://developer.healthvault.com/pages/types/type.aspx?id=30cafccc-047d-4288-94ef-643571f7919d*) has a down-version transform. Through these transforms, HealthVault provides an easy way to move data between an older and newer version of a data type.

Versioning of data types is unique to HealthVault among personal health data platforms. Personal health records are meant to exist over a lifetime, and this feature makes moves seamless from older health items to newer health items.

Other transforms. Transform names containing wpd and hvcc enable the HealthVault Connection Center to convert Windows Portable Device Data to and from HealthVault XML.

Type Schemas

Now that we understand the high-level properties associated with a type and have used the MTT display transform to show the summary of all data types in our application, let's take a closer look at what is entailed in a type's schema, with the specific goal of displaying appropriate values for the Weight type.

Weight is a simple type that scales, and applications can write to or read from it. The XML schema and associated sample representation for this type are shown in Example 4-5.

Example 4-5. XML and schema representation of the HealthVault Weight type

```
Column1:
<schema xmlns:weight="urn:com.microsoft.wc.thing.weight"
    xmlns:t="urn:com.microsoft.wc.thing.types" xmlns:d="urn:com.microsoft.wc.dates"
    xmlns="http://www.w3.org/2001/XMLSchema"
    targetNamespace="urn:com.microsoft.wc.thing.weight">
  <import namespace="urn:com.microsoft.wc.thing.types" schemaLocation="base.xsd" />
  <import namespace="urn:com.microsoft.wc.dates" schemaLocation="dates.xsd" />
  <element name="weight">
    <complexType>
      <sequence>
        <element name="when" minOccurs="1" maxOccurs="1" type="d:date-time">
        </element>
        <element name="value" minOccurs="1" maxOccurs="1" type="t:weight-value">
        </element>
      </sequence>
    </complexType>
  </element>
</schema>

Column2:
<data-xml>
  <weight>
    <when>
      <date>
        <y>1990</y>
        <m>1</m>
        <d>1</d>
      </date>
```

```
    <time>
      <h>1</h>
      <m>0</m>
      <s>0</s>
      <f>0</f>
    </time>
  </when>
  <value>
    <kg>60</kg>
    <display units="lb">132</display>
  </value>
</weight>
<common/>
</data-xml>
```

The Weight type consists of a sequence of date/time and weight values. The use of date/time in HealthVault is defined in the *dates.xsd* schema file (*https://platform.healthvault -ppe.com/platform/XSD/dates.xsd*), and the weight values are defined in the *types.xsd* schema file (*https://platform.healthvault-ppe.com/platform/XSD/types.xsd*).

The HealthVault .NET Web SDK encapsulates a nice object model on top of this XML and gives a user access to Value and When fields, as shown in Figure 4-8.

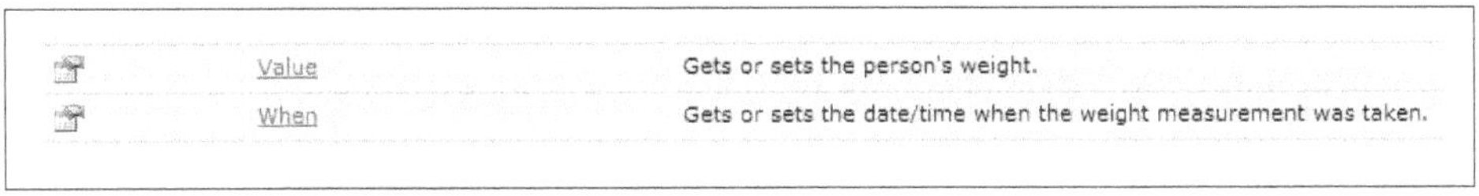

| | Value | Gets or sets the person's weight. |
| | When | Gets or sets the date/time when the weight measurement was taken. |

Figure 4-8. Properties in the HealthVault .NET SDK for the Weight class

Units and measurements

Note that the Value field of this type contains display and units data. HealthVault stores the underlying measurement in kilograms, but the application can show it to the user in the same form in which it was entered. In our example Quantified Self application, we ask the user to input values in pounds. Example 4-6 shows how we convert this value to kilograms for storage while displaying it to the user as pounds (lbs).

Example 4-6. Creating a new Weight value

```
protected void Btn_SubmitWeight_Click(object sender, EventArgs e)
{
    double weight = double.Parse(Txt_Weight.Text);
    Weight w = new Weight(
            new HealthServiceDateTime(DateTime.Now), ❶
            new WeightValue(
                weight * 1.6, new DisplayValue(weight, "lbs", "lbs")));
    w.CommonData.Source = _appName; ❷
    PersonInfo.SelectedRecord.NewItem(w);
}
```

Dates

The When field or date is a special type called `HealthServiceDateTime`. As Line ❶ in Example 4-6 shows, an instance of this date can be created by using the System `Date Time`. HealthVault enables a user to enter varying degrees of date precisions, hence it has a custom date/time.

In fact, the HealthVault approximate datetime construct allows you to create a date as flexible as "when I was a kid" or "Jan 2011" or "Dec". All the different kinds of Health-Vault dates are defined in *dates.xsd*, available at *https://platform.healthvault-ppe.com/ platform/XSD/dates.xsd*.

 One of the core HealthVault design tenets is to ingest all kinds of data. Flexible dates enable a user to enter unstructured data. Furthermore, constructs such as `approx-date-time` allow HealthVault to receive data from standards such as CCR or CCD.

Common data

All types share some common data elements. In Line ❷ of Example 4-6, we are writing to the common data element that shows the source of the application.

Other commonly used data elements are notes, tags, and related items.

Terminologies

HealthVault provides an extensible mechanism to specify strings coded for use across various systems through `codable-value`. The `codable-value` consists of text associated with the code, which is represented in a structured format called `coded-value`.

Terminologies are used in a HealthVault data element called `codable`. This element provides a structured way to represent semantically meaningful text.

Example 4-7 shows a `codable-value` schema. The `family` data field of `coded-value` specifies whether the code belongs to particular code system; for example, `wc` refers to the HealthVault code system, and `HL7` refers to a system adopted by Health Language 7.

Example 4-7. codable-value schema

```
<complexType name="codable-value">
  <sequence>
    <element name="text" type="string">
    </element>
    <element name="code" type="this:coded-value" minOccurs="0" maxOccurs="unbounded">
    </element>
  </sequence>
</complexType>
```

```
<complexType name="coded-value">
  <sequence>
    <element name="value" type="string">
    </element>
    <element name="family" type="string" minOccurs="0">
    </element>
    <element name="type" type="string">
    </element>
    <element name="version" type="string" minOccurs="0">
    </element>
  </sequence>
</complexType>
```

HealthVault has more than 150 terminologies. The wiki *http://partners.mshealthcom munity.com/hv_eco/w/wiki/preferred-vocabularies.aspx* describes how these terminologies are used by the HealthVault user interface, and the book Meaningful Use and Beyond (*http://shop.oreilly.com/product/0636920020110.do*) (Fred Trotter and David Uhlman, O'Reilly) describes how meaningful use, as proposed by federal regulations, dictates the use of these terminologies.

Example 4-8 shows how one can read the Exercise data type for showing calories burned. The Exercise data type stores various kinds of attributes in key value pairs. These attributes are listed in the ExerciseDetail terminology. As Example 4-8 shows, one can use the code value of CaloriesBurned from the ExerciseDetail terminology to look up the appropriate value and display it in the user interface.

Example 4-8. Listing calories burned in the DisplayExercise function

```
private void DisplayExercise(List<Exercise> exercises)
{
    DataTable exercise = new DataTable("exercise");
    exercise.Columns.Add(new DataColumn("Date"));
    exercise.Columns.Add(new DataColumn("ExerciseType"));
    exercise.Columns.Add(new DataColumn("CaloriesBurned"));
    foreach (Exercise e in exercises)
    {
        DataRow row = exercise.NewRow();
        row["Date"] = e.EffectiveDate.ToShortDateString().ToString();
        row["ExerciseType"] = e.Activity.Text;
        if (e.Details.ContainsKey(ExerciseDetail.CaloriesBurned_calories))
        {
            row["CaloriesBurned"] = e.Details[ExerciseDetail.CaloriesBurned_calories];
        }
        exercise.Rows.Add(row);
    }
    ExerciseView.DataSource = exercise;
    ExerciseView.DataBind();
}
```

Extending HealthVault Data Types

Applications frequently have to represent something that is not encapsulated by the data structure of the HealthVault data types. Out of the box, HealthVault provides a mechanism by which a data type can be extended.

Every application can choose to write XML information in the extension tag within the common data section of a data type. It is recommended that applications distinguish their extension elements by using a unique source attribute on the extension element.

In our example, let's assume we are extending the daily dietary intake type to add information on alcohol consumption.

Creating a Type Extension

We would like to track the amount of alcohol consumed in a simple element called "alcoholic-drinks". To simplify things further, we assume this element represents the number of alcoholic drinks including wine, beer, cocktails etc., and is normalized to mean average alcohol per unit.

The first step is to write an alcoholic-drinks XML element within the extension tag using a unique source (_appDailyAlcoholExtensionName) in the extension element. Lines ❶–❷ in Example 4-9 show how one can do it in the .NET SDK.

Example 4-9. Creating a type extension

```
protected void Submit_Daily_Diet_Click(object sender, System.EventArgs e)
{
    //Post Diet
    DietaryDailyIntake diet = new DietaryDailyIntake();
    int totalCarbs;
    int.TryParse(Txt_DailyDietCarbs.Text, out totalCarbs);
    diet.TotalCarbohydrates.Kilograms = totalCarbs * 1000;
    diet.CommonData.Note = Txt_DailyDietNote.Text;

    //Adding extension data
    string drinks = Txt_DailyDietAlcohol.Text;
    HealthRecordItemExtension extension =
        new HealthRecordItemExtension(_appDailyAlcoholExtensionName);
    diet.CommonData.Extensions.Add(extension);
    XPathNavigator navigator = extension.ExtensionData.CreateNavigator(); ❶
    navigator.InnerXml = @"<extension source=""" + _appDailyAlcoholExtensionName + @""">
            <alcoholic-drinks>" + drinks + "</alcoholic-drinks>"; ❷

    PersonInfo.SelectedRecord.NewItem(diet);
}
```

Consuming a Type Extension

The second step is to read information from the extension. In our application, the user enters alcoholic drink information through a text box associated with the Daily Dietary intake section, as shown in Figure 4-9.

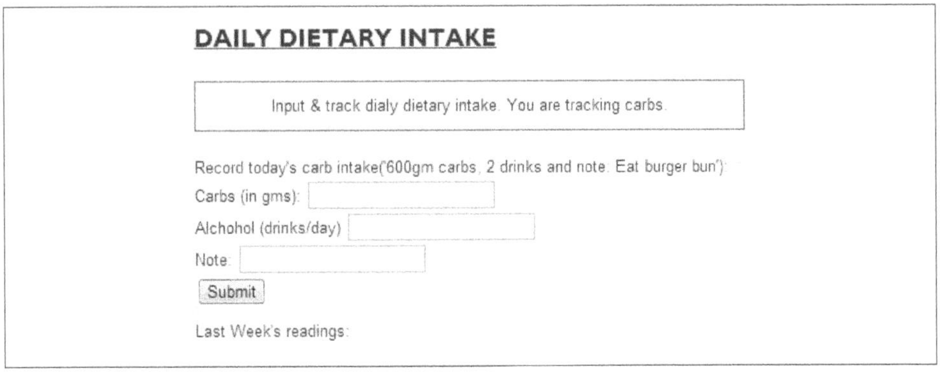

Figure 4-9. Input section for Daily Dietary Intake

Lines ❶–❸ in Example 4-10 show how one can read `<alcoholic-drinks>` XML. To parse this information we use XPath, and in the data type document, the element of interest resides at `extension/alcoholic-drinks`. Using the .NET `XPathNavigator` class, we select a single note signifying this value (Lines ❶–❷). Line ❹ fetches the note associated with this instance of daily dietary intake. The user can potentially input clarifying information—for example, "drank 3 tequila shots"—in this element.

Example 4-10. Consuming a type extension

```
private void DisplayDailyDiet(List<DietaryDailyIntake> dailydiets)
{
    DataTable dailydiet = new DataTable("DailyDiets");
    dailydiet.Columns.Add(new DataColumn("Date"));
    dailydiet.Columns.Add(new DataColumn("Carbs (in gm)"));
    dailydiet.Columns.Add(new DataColumn("Alcohol (#drinks)"));
    dailydiet.Columns.Add(new DataColumn("Note"));
    foreach (DietaryDailyIntake e in dailydiets)
    {
        DataRow row = dailydiet.NewRow();
        row["Date"] = e.EffectiveDate.ToShortDateString().ToString();
        row["Carbs (in gm)"] = e.ToString();
        foreach(HealthRecordItemExtension extension in e.CommonData.Extensions)
        {
            if (extension.Source == _appDailyAlcoholExtensionName)
            {
                XPathNavigator navigator = extension.ExtensionData.CreateNavigator();
                XPathNavigator alcoholicDrinksNavigator = ❶
                    navigator.SelectSingleNode("extension/alcoholic-drinks"); ❷
                if (alcoholicDrinksNavigator != null) ❸
                {
```

```
                row["Alcohol (#drinks)"] = alcoholicDrinksNavigator.Value;
            }
        }
    }
    row["Note"] = e.CommonData.Note;  ❹
    dailydiet.Rows.Add(row);
}
DailyDietView.DataSource = dailydiet;
DailyDietView.DataBind();
}
```

Applications may choose to combine and formalize the two steps just shown and create an extension class, which then could be registered with HealthVault SDK so that every time the extend type is accessed by the application, the appropriate extension properties are available.

Creating Custom Types

Extending a HealthVault data type might not always solve your data needs. Many times there are legitimate use cases for which the application needs a unique data repository. For example, in our Quantified Self application, we need a repository to store all of the user's self-experiments.

HealthVault provides a mechanism called an *application-specific type* for this purpose. This type is not shareable with other applications. Once application developers find a broader use for their data, they can work with Microsoft to create a first-class data type for their needs.

Example 4-11 shows how one can use an application-specific type to store self-experiment hypotheses for the Quantified Self application. In our application we are asking a user to create a hypothesis using a simple text box. The value of this text box is read as the hypothesis string in Line ❶. In Lines ❸–❹, we create an XML document with the data for this specific type and then add it to the document using `Applica tionSpecificXml` in Line ❺. Each application-specific type requires a `SubtypeTag` and `Description` (Lines ❻–❼). We also specify the application creating this type in Line ❷. Additionally, we use the common note element to capture the status of the type in Line ❽, and the `When` element captures the date.

Example 4-11. Writing an application-specific custom type

```
protected void Btn_Submit_Hypothesis_Click(object sender, System.EventArgs e)
{
    ApplicationSpecific appSpecific = new ApplicationSpecific();
    string hypothesis = Txt_Hypothesis.Text;  ❶
    appSpecific.ApplicationId = this.ApplicationConnection.ApplicationId.ToString();  ❷
    XmlDocument xml = new XmlDocument();  ❸
    xml.LoadXml(
        string.Format("<self-experiment><hypothesis>{0}</hypothesis>
            </self-experiment>",
        hypothesis));  ❹
```

```
    appSpecific.ApplicationSpecificXml.Add(xml); ❺
    appSpecific.SubtypeTag = "self-experiment"; ❻
    appSpecific.Description = hypothesis; ❼
    // Default the status note to active when the hypothesis is created
    appSpecific.CommonData.Note = "Active"; ❽
    appSpecific.When = new HealthServiceDateTime(DateTime.Now);
    PersonInfo.SelectedRecord.NewItem(appSpecific);
}
```

On the other hand, we can show the list of self-experiments by reading the `Applica
tionSpecificXml` using an XPath navigator. In Example 4-12, note that in Lines ❶–❷,
we assume that the document for this type contains only one element and that the first
node is the hypothesis.

Example 4-12. Reading an application-specific type

```
private void DisplaySelfExperiments(List<ApplicationSpecific> selfExperiments)
{
    DataTable selfExperiment = new DataTable("SelfExperiments");
    selfExperiment.Columns.Add(new DataColumn("Date"));
    selfExperiment.Columns.Add(new DataColumn("Hypothesis"));
    selfExperiment.Columns.Add(new DataColumn("Status"));
    foreach (ApplicationSpecific s in selfExperiments)
    {

        DataRow row = selfExperiment.NewRow();
        row["Date"] = s.EffectiveDate.ToShortDateString().ToString();
        row["Hypothesis"] = s.ApplicationSpecificXml[0].CreateNavigator(). ❶
                            SelectSingleNode("hypothesis").Value; ❷
        row["Status"] = s.CommonData.Note;
        selfExperiment.Rows.Add(row);
    }
    SelfExperimentsView.DataSource = selfExperiment;
    SelfExperimentsView.DataBind();
}
```

Trusting Data in HealthVault Data Types

Knowing the origin of data is often critical for an application that is using it for sensitive
purposes. Some use cases warrant working with only trusted data, some warrant knowing whether the data is from a device or self-entered by the users, and in some cases the
application might just want to work with known data providers.

HealthVault provides several ways to look at data provenance. Applications can look
at the `created_by` and `updated_by` fields of a data type and see whether they were updated
by devices or known applications. Additionally, HealthVault provides digital signing
of data, which can create a very secure ecosystem of trust.

In our example, we look at the `Source` attribute of Weight items to see whether they
were uploaded by a Withings scale or added manually by the user.

Digitally Signing Data

HealthVault provides a way to digitally sign all data types. For instance, using the .NET SDK, an application can sign HealthVault types very easily. Example 4-13 shows a snippet of code that can be used to sign the Weight data type. The certificate in **cert.Import** can be obtained from a trusted provider such as VeriSign, Comodo, etc.

Example 4-13. Signing Weight data

```
protected void Btn_SubmitAndSignWeight_Click(object sender, EventArgs e)
{
  double weight = double.Parse(Txt_Weight.Text);
  Weight w = new Weight(
      new HealthServiceDateTime(DateTime.Now),
      new WeightValue(
        weight * 1.6, new DisplayValue(weight, "lbs", "lbs")));

  X509Certificate2 cert = new X509Certificate2();
  cert.Import("..\\cert\valid_cert.pfx");

  w.Sign(cert);
  PersonInfo.SelectedRecord.NewItem(w);

}
```

The verification of a digitally signed certificate is available through the **IsSignatureValid()** and **ValidateCertificate()** methods in the HealthVault .NET SDK.

In the samples associated with this chapter (*ThingSignatureSample.java*), you can review the code for doing digital signing of HealthVault data types using the HealthVault Java library.

Relating HealthVault Data Types

HealthVault data types are intended to be self-contained units of health information. The data types have distinct health items, such as medications, immunizations, and weight readings. This approach is characteristically different from relational data modeling in which the data is normalized and stored in distinct tables that have explicit relationships with each other. For example, in a relational model, medications may be expressed as separate medication name and medication dosage tables.

Often there is a need to represent relationships between individual health items. For example, a Medication is inherently related to Medication Fill. Medications are associated with a person's profile as prescribed by a physician, and Medication Fill is used by a pharmacy to prescribe units of medications to a consumer as she consumes the prescribed medications.

The relationship between Medication and Medication Fill is expressed by *related items*. HealthVault offers related items as an inherent mechanism to link and associate data types. A related item is a special chunk of XML that resides in the common data of a health item. Relationships are usually described in the dependent item and link to the more independent one. For instance, to express the relationship between Medication Fill and Medication, one places related items in the Medication Fill type and points to the Medication type.

Another interesting use of related items is to link together a set of readings that are uploaded from a single device. For example, a device calculating body fat percentage and cholesterol can associate them through related items while uploading them. Because this association is done before uploading to HealthVault, a special unique identifier called a client ID can be used. Client IDs are usually unique identifiers associated to instances of HealthVault data types and are created by the client uploading the data.

One can take relationships even further and associate a set of medical images, medications, and conditions as a result of a particular health incident, maybe an accident. The Mayo Clinic Health Manager application provides a way to create a web of related HealthVault items.

Related items lie beyond the scope of this book, but the reader is encouraged to explore them and contribute interesting uses and examples at *http://enablingprogrammableself.com*.

Exploring HealthVault Data Types

In our example, we picked some HealthVault types to be used in the application based on our device, data availability, and purpose. Every application programmer needs to go through this data exploration based on your needs and goals. This section gives an overview of all HealthVault types so that the reader can have a good understanding of what is available in the system.

Categorizing HealthVault Data Types

HealthVault stores personal health information ranging from fitness data to medical images. Table 4-1 shows the categorization of the data as displayed to the end user.

Table 4-1. End user categorization of HealthVault data

Category	HealthVault types
Fitness	Aerobic Exercise Session, Aerobic Profile, Aerobic Weekly Goal, Calorie Guideline, Daily Dietary Intake, Exercise, Exercise Samples, Weight Goal
Conditions	Allergy, Concern, Condition, Contraindication, Emotional State, Pregnancy, Problem, Respiratory Profile
Medications	Asthma Inhaler, Asthma Inhaler Use, Daily Medication Usage, Insulin Injection, Insulin Injection Use, Medication, Medication Fill
Health History	Allergic Episode, Annotation, Cardiac Profile, Diabetic Profile, Discharge Summary, Encounter, Explanation of Benefits, Family History, Family History Condition, Family History Person, Health Assessment, Immunization, Procedure, Question Answer

Category	HealthVault types
Measurements	Blood Glucose, Blood Oxygen Saturation, Blood Pressure, Body Composition, Body Dimension, Cholesterol Profile, Device, Genetic SNP Results, HbA1C, Heart Rate, Height, Lab Test Results, Microbiology Lab Results, PAP Session, Peak Flow, Radiology Lab Results, Sleep Journal AM, Sleep Journal PM, Spirometer, Vital Signs, Weight
Personal Profile	Advance Directive, Appointment, Basic, Contact, Healthcare Proxy, Life Goal, Payer, Person (emergency or provider contact), Personal Demographic Information, Personal Image
Files	Clinical Document Architecture (CDA), Continuity of Care Document (CCD), Continuity of Care Record (CCR), File, Medical Image Study, Password-Protected Package
Custom Data	Application Data Reference, Application Specific, Group Membership, Group Membership Activity, Link, Status

Fitness

HealthVault offers a range of fitness types. The most commonly used fitness data type is Exercise. Exercise provides a terminology-based categorization of kinds of exercise, e.g., walking or running. Each activity can also be associated with terminology-driven units: Count, Mile, etc.

Devices such as FitBit and Withings work with this type. The exercise activities terminology lists a range of exercise values, including running, walking, swimming, etc. Devices that fetch detailed information on exercise can write individual samples to the Exercise Sample type. For instance, exercise watches developed by Polar write to exercise samples in addition to summarizing the workout in the Exercise type.

This category of types is implemented in a fairly generic way so that various industry formats, such as the one used by Garmin's Connect website (*http://connect.garmin.com/*), can translate easily to these types. ISO units can also be translated easily to HealthVault units.

Conditions

Health problems, allergies, contra-indications, and mental health (emotional state) are categorized in the Condition set of types. Conditions are sensitive health problems that usually have an onset date and a status associated with them.

The HealthVault Shell uses the Condition type to record conditions. Conditions entered through the user interface are mapped to SNOMED-CT terminology.

Medication

Medications are the center of modern medicine. HealthVault offers a number of granular types to capture the essence of medications.

A number of pharmacies, including CVS and Walgreens, offer applications for importing prescription data into HealthVault, but the user interface and integration for these applications is a bit challenging.

The most frequently used data types in this category are Medication and Medication Fill. Each prescription could be broken into Medication and Medication Fill. Medication Fill is the recurring part of one's prescription. As you may recall from "Relating HealthVault Data Types" on page 70, the Medication Fill type is usually related to Medication using the related-item semantics when entered through the HealthVault Shell.

Medications are mapped or coded to the RxNorm Active Medicines terminology.

Health History

Immunizations, procedures, family history, health events, etc. form the basis of the Health History category.

The most notable application using types in this category is the Surgeon General's Family History application (*https://familyhistory.hhs.gov/fhh-web*). This powerful application enables individuals to easily create a family health history tree.

Measurements

Measurements are the most extensive category of HealthVault data types. Measurements range from the output of various fitness devices to lab results. For instance, the Withings weighing scale writes to the weight measures, and FitBit writes to sleep measures. The measures are granular records of daily activity and consequently are traceable.

On the other hand, the Lab Test Results type, one of the most complicated HealthVault types, represents results from labs. It can be used in conjunction with industry-standard terminologies.

Personal Profile

The Personal Profile category of HealthVault types contains data pertaining to health care proxies, personal images, and demographics. Almost every HealthVault application that shows a user's picture or looks at ages or other demographic information uses types in this category.

Files

HealthVault, unlike most personal health records, allows you to upload a number of types of files, and therefore supports data types for these files. Example 4-14 shows the file extensions supported, displayed through a `GetServiceDefinition` call in Power-Shell. This information can also be viewed online in the HealthVault Developer Center's service definition section (*http://developer.healthvault.com/pages/methods/methods.aspx*).

Example 4-14. List of file extensions supported by HealthVault

```
PS C:\Windows\system32> $a = Get-ServiceDefinition
PS C:\Windows\system32> $a.ConfigurationValues

Key                            Value
---                            -----
allowedDocumentExtensions      .avi,.bluebutton,.bmp,.ccd,.ccr,.cda,.doc,.docm,...
autoReconcilableTypes          1e1ccbfc-a55d-4d91-8940-fa2fbf73c195,9c48a2b8-...
blobHashBlockSizeBytes         2097152
blobHashDefaultAlgorithm       SHA256Block
blobStreamWriteTokenTtlMs      172800000
defaultCulture                 en
defaultPersonInfosPerRetrieval 200
emailValidationExp             ^([\w-+\.]+)@((\[[0-9]{1,3}\.[0-9]{1,3}\.[0-9]...
liveIdAuthPolicy               HBI
liveIdEnvironment              PROD
<... clipped for brevity..>
```

The Medical Image study type used by the HealthVault Connection Center uploads DICOM medical images in this type. The CCD/CCR types are industry-standard ways by which various hospital information systems send care records to HealthVault. Google Health users, for instance, migrated to HealthVault using the CCR type. The Message file type is the backbone of HealthVault's Direct integration. Any email message received by the user is stored in the Message type.

Custom Data

The Application Specific type, already covered in the section "Creating Custom Types" on page 68 with regard to adding a repository in which to store self-experiments, is the most important custom data type. This type is used by various applications to store information in HealthVault for which no other type or extension to a type is appropriate. For instance, the Vivacity's Spending Scout application (*http://www.spen dingscout.com/*) stored explanation of benefit information in this type until the Health-Vault team created an Explanation of Benefits (EOB) type to support it more directly.

Contributing to the Self-Experimentation Application

In next chapter we will see how we can augment the self-experimentation web application by creating mobile applications. The source for the application is available at *http://enablingprogrammableself.com*, and we are inviting you, dear reader, to extend this application and make it your own. Perhaps fork the Git repository and contribute your code back, or create Java, Ruby, or Python versions of it!

CHAPTER 5

Enabling mHealth for Quantified Self

"Think: mHealth as personal health reform."

—Jane Sarasohn-Kahn

Having an accessible and programmable health record sets HealthVault apart. It enables a rich ecosystem of devices and mobile and web applications. Chapter 3 focused on introducing the HealthVault API, and Chapter 4 gave a good overview of Health-Vault data types using a data-intensive Quantified Self application. This chapter takes a closer look at building mobile applications for HealthVault.

We will look at an end-to-end example of building a mood-tracking application on top of mobile platforms. The chapter will cover elements of mobile client programming using code samples for Windows Phone 7 (C#). Similar interfaces are available for Android (Java) and iOS (Objective-C).

The Mood Tracker Mobile Application

In Chapter 3, we built an end-to-end web application that enables a user to track several kinds of data and use that data to help with self-experimentation. Many elements of self-tracking data, such as sleep, weight, and exercise, have the capability to be measured through devices; however, it's very hard to measure elements of happiness, such as mood and stress, automatically.

In recent years, we have seen a surge in mobile smartphone devices. Mobile devices offer a very effective tool for efficient data entry and are an ideal platform to build data collection tools. So our manual "mood tracking" need could be served by an application that makes it easy and engaging for a user to track mood using a smartphone. For the purposes of our example, let's build the application on the Windows Phone 7 platform.

So, What Should We Build?

The application will allow the user to input his mood, well-being, and stress level; present a way to look at the history of the data; and add a bit of zest using a "mood plant" avatar. The mood plant summarizes the user's emotional state over time. When the user is happy, stress-free, and fit for a long time, the plant thrives, showing a happy face (☺), and in the case of depression and stress, it shows the effects of bad health (☹).

Figure 5-1 is a sketch of what the app might look like.

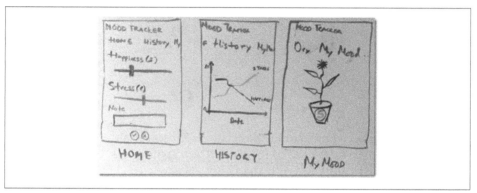

Figure 5-1. White board wire-frame of our mood tracking application

Choosing HealthVault Integration

The first question we need to answer is what kind of HealthVault connectivity this application requires. We discussed several models of connecting with HealthVault in Chapter 3. As this application is only for a client device, we will use a client application model and the HealthVault Windows Phone 7 client library. Having a client application allows you to provide a rich interface and the potential capability to store the readings locally.

Selecting Appropriate HealthVault Data Types

The next question we should solve is which HealthVault data types to use. We discussed HealthVault data types in detail in Chapter 4. Various data types could apply in this context, but browsing the HealthVault data types (*http://developer.healthvault .com/pages/types/types.aspx*) reveals one relevant data type in particular: Emotional State (*http://developer.healthvault.com/pages/types/type.aspx?id=4b7971d6-e427-427d -bf2c-2fbcf76606b3*).

On further analysis, it turns out that this type is almost perfect for our use. Mood, stress, and well-being are rated on a scale of 1–5. We do a further reading of associations for each of these values, and add appropriate textual elements for each of the values (mood, stress, and well-being).

Getting Started

I assume you have Visual Studio installed with Window Phone 7 (WP7) tools. If not, you can get them from *http://create.msdn.com/en-us/home/getting_started*.

Next, go over to CodePlex (*http://healthvaultwp7.codeplex.com/*) at *http://health vaultwp7.codeplex.com/* and download the HealthVault library with sample applications.

I extracted the library to my desktop, and the folder structure looks like Figure 5-2. *HvMobileRegular* has the relevant C# code to abstract for working with the Health-Vault web service, and *HvMobilePhone* uses the code in *HvMobileRegular* to build a library that works with Windows Phone 7 platform. The *TestRegular* directory has a unit test for the HealthVault mobile Windows Phone 7 (WP7) library. *WeightTrackerDemo* is a sample application that shows use cases of the library for a Weight Tracking application.

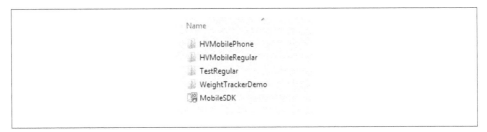

Figure 5-2. HealthVault WP7 library extracted

If you open the MobileSDK solution in Visual Studio and press F5, the library compiles and the WeightTracker demo starts. Figure 5-3 shows this application in action; we will use this application as a template for building ours.

Without further ado, let's create our new Silverlight for Windows Phone project. We can create a solution for MoodTracker and reference the *HVMobilePhone* library in that project. You can also use the existing project, MobileSDK, and associate a new application in it; in the source code associated with this chapter, I created a new project called MoodTracker (Figure 5-4).

First things first: let's set up the application to talk to HealthVault. In the *App.xaml.cs* class, add a reference to the HealthVault Service and HealthVault Shell. We also need to make sure we get a unique application ID in the developer environment of HealthVault. To do that, we head over to the HealthVault Application Configuration Center (*http://config.healthvault-ppe.com/*) and create a new application by clicking on the "Create a new application" button (Figure 5-5). Note that in Chapter 3 we used the Application Manager utility to create a web application, but in this chapter we use an alternative method that allows us to create client applications as well as web applications.

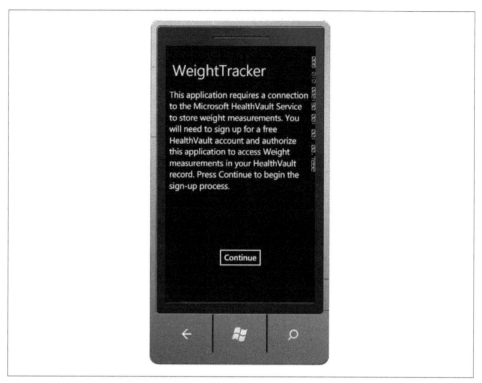

Figure 5-3. Compiling and running the HealthVault WP7 sample application

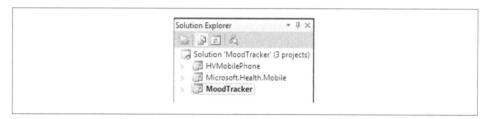

Figure 5-4. Beginnings of Mood Tracker

We create an application of type Software on Device Auth (SODA), which is an authentication mechanism for client applications, and pick the name Mood Tracker for it, as shown in Figure 5-6.

Once the application is created, we need to assign appropriate authorization rules for the data types that the application will access. To do that, click on the app's link and assign appropriate data types for the application, as shown in Figure 5-7.

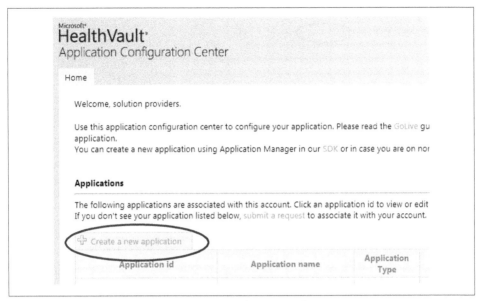

Figure 5-5. Creating a new application in the Application Configuration Center

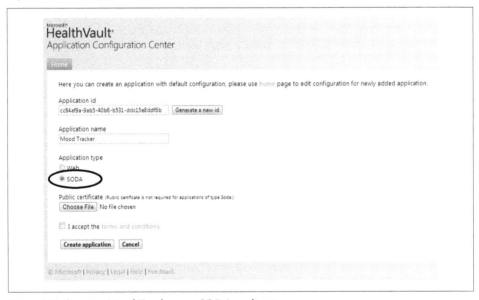

Figure 5-6. Creating Mood Tracker as a SODA application

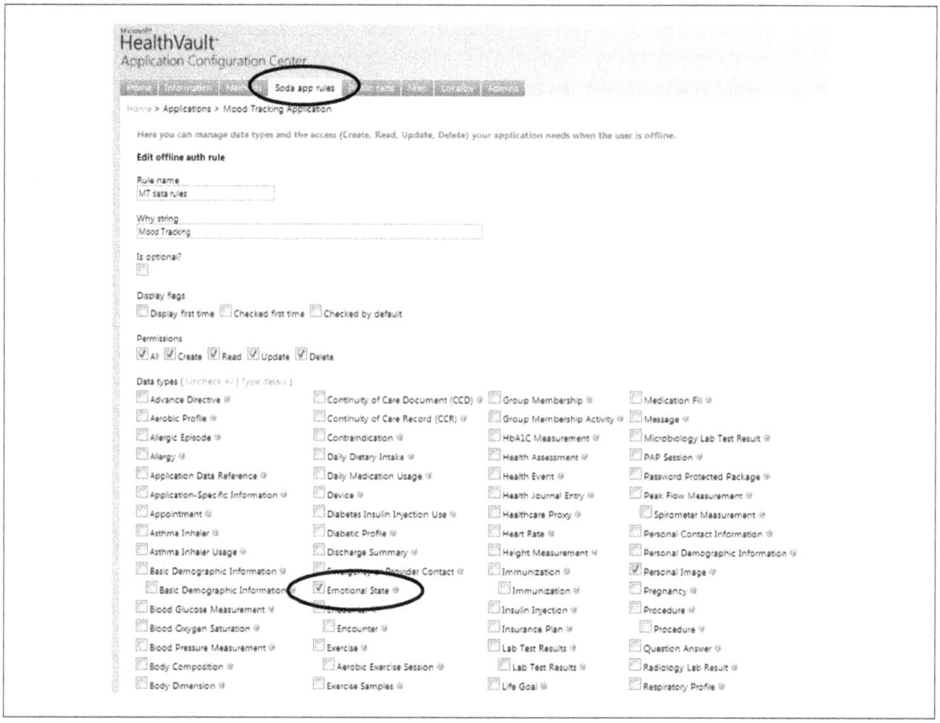

Figure 5-7. Adding Emotional State to our Mood Tracker application

Having created the client application and assigned data type authorization rules, we are all set! Now let's configure the base page to work with the HealthVault preproduction environment (PPE). The PPE is the development environment publicly available for all HealthVault developers. The HealthVault platform in this environment is available at *https://platform.healthvault-ppe.com/platform/wildcat.ashx*, and the Health-Vault shell in this environment is available at *https://account.healthvault.com*. Chapter 6 will show how to deploy your app to the general public after you have developed and tested it.

Example 5-1 shows the initial code for configuring the application. In Line ❶, we assign the `platformUrl`; in Line ❷, we assign the `shellUrl`; and Line ❸ is the application identifier that we created using the Application Configuration Center. The `HealthVaultSer vice` object initialized the HealthVault Windows Phone 7 library with appropriate configuration variables. Using this object, we can make all the relevant HealthVault web service requests.

Example 5-1. Configuring the client application

```
namespace MoodTracker
{
    public partial class App : Application
    {
```

```
public static string SettingsFilename = "Settings";
public static HealthVaultService HealthVaultService { get; set; }
public static string HealthVaultShellUrl { get; set; }

static string platformUrl =
    @"https://platform.healthvault-ppe.com/platform/wildcat.ashx"; ❶
static string shellUrl = @"https://account.healthvault-ppe.com"; ❷
static string masterAppId = "83bf507d-9186-407f-a6cd-b2d65f558690"; ❸

// Code to execute when the application is launching (eg, from Start)
// This code will not execute when the application is reactivated
private void Application_Launching(object sender, LaunchingEventArgs e)
{
    HealthVaultService = new HealthVaultService
        (platformUrl, shellUrl, new Guid(masterAppId));
}
// Code to execute when the application is activated (brought to foreground)
// This code will not execute when the application is first launched
private void Application_Activated(object sender, ActivatedEventArgs e)
{
    HealthVaultService = new HealthVaultService
        (platformUrl, shellUrl, new Guid(masterAppId));
}
```

We can make this project a startup project, press F5, and get to the first page of our application. We're in business!

Authenticating the Application and User with HealthVault

In order for the Mood Tracker application to work with HealthVault, we will get appropriate application creation credentials from the HealthVault Service. We must also set up a method by which the user can authorize the application using the HealthVault Shell.

1. To get the credentials from the HealthVault Service, the application contacts the HealthVault service to get an application creation URL. The code for that is outlined in *MyMood.xaml.cs* (*https://github.com/vaibhavb/moodtracker/blob/master/MoodTracker/MyMood.xaml.cs*) (Example 5-2).

    Example 5-2. Authenticating the application with HealthVaultService

    ```
    void MainPage_Loaded(object sender, RoutedEventArgs e)
    {
        App.HealthVaultService.LoadSettings(App.SettingsFilename);
        App.HealthVaultService.BeginAuthenticationCheck(AuthenticationCompleted,
            DoShellAuthentication);
        SetProgressBarVisibility(true);
    }

    void DoShellAuthentication(object sender, HealthVaultResponseEventArgs e)
    {
        SetProgressBarVisibility(false);
    ```

```
App.HealthVaultService.SaveSettings(App.SettingsFilename);

string url;

if (_addingRecord)
{
    url = App.HealthVaultService.GetUserAuthorizationUrl();
}
else
{
    url = App.HealthVaultService.GetApplicationCreationUrl();
}
```

2. The application creation needs to be validated on behalf of the user.

The best mechanism to achieve this is by having a page with a hosted browser that redirects appropriately to HealthVault, and then closes the browser and navigates back to the application page after a successful authorization.

Example 5-3 is the relevant code in *HostedBrowserPage.xaml*.

Example 5-3. Using a hosted browser to show HealthVault user authentication

```
void c_webBrowser_Navigated
    (object sender, System.Windows.Navigation.NavigationEventArgs e)
{
    if (e.Uri.OriginalString.Contains("target=AppAuthSuccess"))
    {
        Uri pageUri = new Uri("/MyMood.xaml", UriKind.RelativeOrAbsolute);

        Deployment.Current.Dispatcher.BeginInvoke(() =>
        {
            NavigationService.Navigate(pageUri);
        });
    }
}

void HealthVaultWebPage_Loaded(object sender, RoutedEventArgs e)
{
    string url = App.HealthVaultShellUrl;

    c_webBrowser.Navigate(new Uri(url));
}
```

Note that on success, the application is redirected to *MyMood.xaml*, which is our application's landing page.

Figure 5-8 shows the flow of how the authentication described here works.

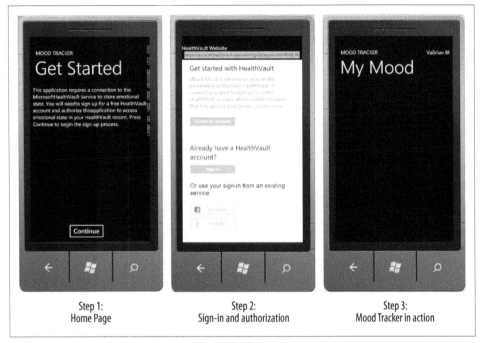

Step 1:
Home Page

Step 2:
Sign-in and authorization

Step 3:
Mood Tracker in action

Figure 5-8. Authentication model with HealthVault

Reading Data from HealthVault

The data type we settled on for our application was Emotional State. Our first goal is to be able to read data for this type and display it in our application. To do this, we need test data for emotional state. Add test information into the test or developer account for this application from the list of type samples (*http://developer.healthvault .com/pages/types/types.aspx*) associated with the Emotional State type in the Health-Vault Developer Center (*http://developer.healthvault.com/pages/types/types.aspx*), as shown in Figure 5-9. An important thing to note is that you need to be signed into *http: //developer.healthvault.com* to add the sample; otherwise, this application gives an error.

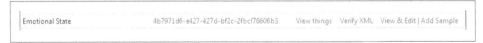

Figure 5-9. Adding an Emotional State sample to HealthVault record

We can verify that this sample is added to our record by viewing the information in the HealthVault PPE shell interface (*https://account.healthvault-ppe.com*), as shown in Figure 5-10.

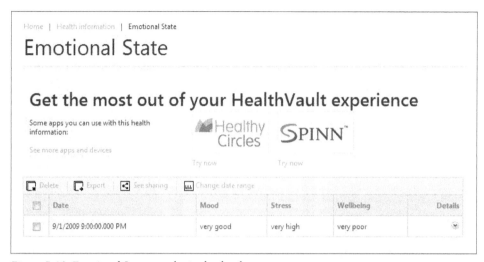

Emotional State

Get the most out of your HealthVault experience

Some apps you can use with this health
information:

See more apps and devices

Healthy Circles

SPINN™

Try now   Try now

	Date	Mood	Stress	Wellbeing	Details
	9/1/2009 9:00:00.000 PM	very good	very high	very poor	⌄

Delete   Export   See sharing   Change date range

Figure 5-10. Emotional State samples in the developer account

Chapter 2 explained the HealthVault `GetThings` method. This method enables an application to read data from the user's health record. A read request for health data can be performed using various querying mechanisms. For the purposes of this application, we will retrieve the last active item for the user's Emotional State data type (Example 5-4).

Example 5-4. Using GetThings

```
HealthVaultMethods.GetThings
    (EmotionalStateModel.TypeId, 1, null, null, GetThingsCompleted);
```

To make it easier to work with GetThings, I implemented a simple abstraction on the method in the `HealthVaultMethods` class. Example 5-5 shows the code for this abstraction. It allows the construction of a GetThings query for one type ID, with the maximum items returned and with the appropriate minimum and maximum effective dates for these health items. Chapter 4 explains the XML query sent by the `GetThings` method in detail.

Example 5-5. GetThings abstraction

```
        public static void GetThings(string typeId,
            int? maxItems,
            DateTime? effDateMin,
            DateTime? effDateMax,
            EventHandler<HealthVaultResponseEventArgs> responseCallback)
        {
            string thingXml = @"
            <info>
                <group {0}>
                    <filter>
                        <type-id>{1}</type-id>
```

```
                    <thing-state>Active</thing-state>
                    {2}
                    {3}
                </filter>
                <format>
                    <section>core</section>
                    <xml/>
                    <type-version-format>{1}</type-version-format>
                </format>
            </group>
        </info>";

        XElement info = XElement.Parse(string.Format
            (thingXml,
            MaxItemsXml(maxItems),
            typeId,
            EffDateMinXml(effDateMin),
            EffDateMaxXml(effDateMax)));
        HealthVaultRequest request = new HealthVaultRequest
            ("GetThings", "3", info, responseCallback);
        App.HealthVaultService.BeginSendRequest(request);
    }
```

Now, once we can get Emotional State things, we need to perform two action things on the client side.

First, pick the item we are interested in from the GetThings response. To choose the appropriate item, LINQ to XML comes in very handy, offering a SQL-like select clause for XML data, as shown in Example 5-6. LINQ stands for Language Integrated Querying, and it allows for making queries natively from C#.

Example 5-6. Choosing things from a GetThings response

```
// using LINQ to get the latest reading of emotional state
XElement latestEmotion = (from thingNode in responseNode.Descendants("thing")
                                     orderby Convert.ToDateTime(thingNode.Element
                                         ("eff-date").Value) descending
                                     select thingNode).FirstOrDefault<XElement>();
```

Second, parse the items returned for mood, stress, and well-being data. We can achieve this by creating a model for Emotional State. This model is available for review in the *EmotionalStateModel.cs* file. The parse method in this model parses the appropriate elements in thingXml. Chapter 4 details the format of this XML. Notice that in Line ❷ of Example 5-7, we parse the common element to fetch the note data for the Emotional State type. In Line ❶, we are setting the When date of the instance to the eff-date element. We have created enumerations for Mood, Stress, and Wellbeing values, and we can parse the integers for those values using the Enum.Parse method.

Example 5-7. Parsing a thing for the Emotion State data type

```
public void Parse(XElement thingXml)
{
    this.Mood = Mood.None;
    this.Stress = Stress.None;
    this.Wellbeing = Wellbeing.None;

    XElement emotionalState = thingXml.Descendants
        ("data-xml").Descendants("emotion").First();

    this.When = Convert.ToDateTime(thingXml.Element("eff-date").Value); ❶

    if (thingXml.Descendants("common") != null && ❷
            (thingXml.Descendants("common").Descendants("note").Count() != 0))
    {
      this.Note = thingXml.Descendants("common").Descendants("note").First().Value;
    }

    if (emotionalState.Element("mood") != null)
    {
        try
        {
            this.Mood = (Mood)System.Enum.Parse(typeof(Mood),
                ((XElement)emotionalState.Element("mood")).Value, true);
        }
        catch (Exception) { }
    }
    if (emotionalState.Element("stress") != null)
    {
        try
        {
            this.Stress = (Stress)System.Enum.Parse(typeof(Stress),
                ((XElement)emotionalState.Element("stress")).Value, true);
        }
        catch (Exception) { }
    }
    if (emotionalState.Element("wellbeing") != null)
    {
        try
        {
            this.Wellbeing = (Wellbeing)System.Enum.Parse(typeof(Wellbeing),
            ((XElement)emotionalState.Element("wellbeing")).Value, true);
        }
        catch (Exception) { }
    }
}
```

After retrieving the data in our Emotional State model, we can use XAML to view it in our application. XAML is the user interface markup technology for Windows Phone 7. For the purposes of this book, we won't go into the details of XAML. Figure 5-11 shows the display of the latest emotional state reading from HealthVault.

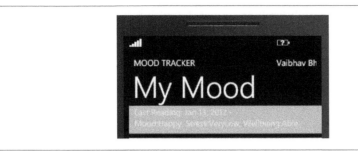

Figure 5-11. Latest Emotional State reading in Mood Tracker!

Writing Data to HealthVault

In the previous section we discussed how one can display the data retrieved from the HealthVault Emotional State data type. Before we get to the topic of this section and discuss how we can put new items into HealthVault, Figure 5-12 shows a screenshot of how the application looks once we have enabled the put.

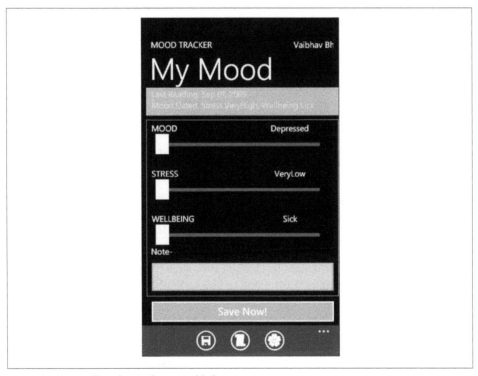

Figure 5-12. MoodTracker with put enabled

For each of the emotional states—mood, stress, and well-being—we have a slider that lets users capture their emotional state. They can also add a note pertaining to their moods using a text box. We want this information to be uploaded with the current time stamp once the user hits the Save Now! button.

Example 5-8 shows how the save button submits information to HealthVault. Note that in Line ❶ we are calling an abstraction for the PutThings method.

Example 5-8. Saving new data to HealthVault

```
// Save the reading to HealthVault
private void Btn_SaveReadingToHealthVault_Click(object sender, RoutedEventArgs e)
{
    EmotionalStateModel model = new EmotionalStateModel();
    model.Mood = (Mood)c_MoodSlider.Value;
    model.Stress = (Stress)c_StressSlider.Value;
    model.Wellbeing = (Wellbeing)c_WellbeingSlider.Value;
    model.When = DateTime.Now;
    model.Note = GetNote();
    HealthVaultMethods.PutThings(model, PutThingsCompleted); ❶
    SetProgressBarVisibility(true);
}
```

In Chapter 3, we looked at the PutThings method in detail. This method enables an application to add or update health items in a user's record. As the first line in Example 5-9 shows, our abstraction fetches the relevant information from the base health record item object and submits that to HealthVault using the PutThings version 2 API. The response for this request is handled by the responseCallback function, which in turn can check for various return codes from the service.

Example 5-9. PutThings abstraction

```
public static void PutThings(HealthRecordItemModel item,
    EventHandler<HealthVaultResponseEventArgs> responseCallback)
{
    XElement info = XElement.Parse(item.GetXml());
    HealthVaultRequest request = new HealthVaultRequest
        ("PutThings", "2", info, responseCallback);
    App.HealthVaultService.BeginSendRequest(request);
}
```

Now that we are able to write data to HealthVault, we have a mobile application that can read and update information from and to HealthVault!

Graphing Mood

In the last section, we enabled Mood Tracker (*http://healthblog.vitraag.com/2011/06/ entering-new-data-with-mood-tracker-5/*) to enter new data in HealthVault. We want to be able to discover patterns in mood, stress, and well-being, and graphing them over time is a great mechanism by which to achieve this goal. Let's start with a simplistic approach, showing the Emotional State readings for mood, stress, and well-being over a week. As Figure 5-13 shows, a user can browse mood readings based on a weekly margin and move forward or backward a week at time.

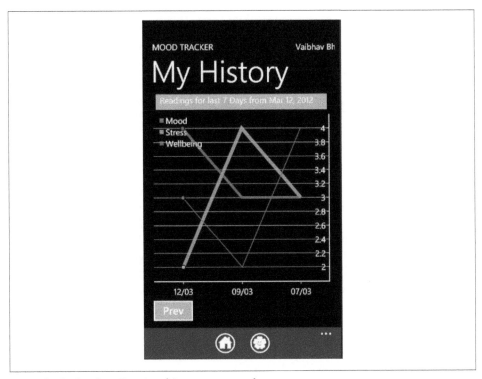

Figure 5-13. Graphing Emotional State over seven days

In order to get data from HealthVault for a specific time period, the GetThings method (*https://github.com/vaibhavb/moodtracker/blob/master/MoodTracker/HealthVaultMe thods.cs*) needs to have the effective date filter enabled to look for appropriate readings. Line ❶ in Example 5-10 shows how the GetThings abstraction is configured to return elements for the last seven days only.

Example 5-10. Fetching readings for the last seven days

```
void RefreshGraph()
{
    this.EmotionList.Clear();
    this.GraphLabel.Text = string.Format("Readings for last 7 Days from {0}",
        BaseTimeForGraph.ToString("MMM dd, yyyy"));
    // Get the last emotional state info and try to plot a graph
    HealthVaultMethods.GetThings(EmotionalStateModel.TypeId, null,
        BaseTimeForGraph.Subtract(new TimeSpan(7, 0, 0, 0)), ❶
        BaseTimeForGraph,
        GetThingsCompleted);
}
```

Note that the `eff-date-min` element, as implemented in the GetThings class in *Health-VautlMethods.cs*, must be formatted in the ISO 8601 format. Line ❶ in Example 5-11 shows how we do the formatting.

Example 5-11. Formatting eff-date-min for the GetThings request

```
private static string EffDateMinXml(DateTime? effDateMin)
{
    if (effDateMin != null)
        return
            string.Format(@"<eff-date-min>{0}</eff-date-min>", ❶
                effDateMin.Value.ToString("yyyy-MM-ddTHH:mm:ss.FFFZ",
                            CultureInfo.InvariantCulture)
            );
    else return "";
}
```

Once we can selectively get information from HealthVault, we can use a graphing library to show the readings. In our case, I chose the open source graphing library am-Charts based on its ease of use. In fact, I added it to the project with one click using the NuGet package manager (*http://www.nuget.org/packages/amChartsQuickCharts*). Example 5-12 shows a snippet of the configuration code showing how the graph is set up for mood, stress, and well-being using a serial chart. Note that the series values are bound in Line ❶ using a `DataSource` called `EmotionList`; it is a list of *observable* emotional states.

Example 5-12. Graphing emotional state

```
<amq:SerialChart x:Name="EmotionsChart"
            BorderThickness="1"
            DataSource="{Binding EmotionList}" ❶
            CategoryValueMemberPath="FormattedWhen"
            AxisForeground="White"
            PlotAreaBackground="Black"
            GridStroke="DarkGray" Height="463" Width="450">
    <amq:SerialChart.Graphs>
        <amq:LineGraph ValueMemberPath="Mood"
                    Title="Mood" Brush="Blue"
                    StrokeThickness="6"
                    BorderBrush="Cornsilk"/>
        <amq:LineGraph ValueMemberPath="Stress"
                    Title="Stress" Brush="#8000FF00"
                    StrokeThickness="8" />
        <amq:LineGraph ValueMemberPath="Wellbeing"
                    Title="Wellbeing"
                    StrokeThickness="2"
                    Brush="#80FF0000"/>
    </amq:SerialChart.Graphs>
</amq:SerialChart>
```

Data Analysis: Mood Plant

We want a user to engage with the emotional state readings, and a good way to achieve this goal is by providing a zestful visualization for their emotional state. We use a mood plant as a mechanism to gauge a user's emotional state over the recent past.

The flower of the plant represents the average mood, the leaves represent average stress, and the roots represent the average well-being. Individual flower, leaf, and root ligatures map the values 0 through 5 to mood, stress, and well-being. The final mood plant is a result of superimposing these values. Figure 5-14 shows an instance of a mood plant with mood 3, stress 3, and well-being 3.

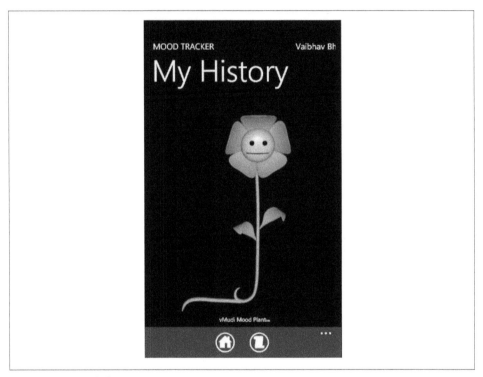

Figure 5-14. Mood plant

So how do we find average mood, stress, or well-being? Various correlations and algorithms can be used to express the average emotional state over time. We will start with a simple function that creates an average mood, stress, or well-being score based on a weighted average of the values. The function takes the readings for mood, stress, or well-being for the past month and assigns a 50% weight to the most recent week, 30% to week 3, and 20% to weeks 1 and 2 of the month's readings. It is left as an exercise to the reader to evaluate and try different functions. Example 5-13 shows the code for the weighting algorithm.

Example 5-13. Algorithm for calculating mood, stress, and well-being over the past month

```
/*
 * Algorithm
 * 1. Read last 1 month's readings
 * 2. Weight 50% to 4th week
 * 3. Weight 25% to 1-3 week
 * 4. Weight 25% to how many readings (Good is 4/wk)
 */
DateTime time50p = baseTime.Subtract(new TimeSpan(7,0,0,0));
DateTime time30p = baseTime.Subtract(new TimeSpan(14, 0, 0, 0));

int m = 0; int s = 0; int w = 0;
int c50 = 0; int c30 = 0; int c20 = 0;
foreach (EmotionalStateModel emotion in emotionList)
{
    if (emotion.When >= time50p)
    {
        m += (int)emotion.Mood * 50 ;
        s += (int)emotion.Stress * 50 ;
        w += (int)emotion.Wellbeing * 50;
        c50++;
    }
    else if (emotion.When >= time30p)
    {
        m += (int)emotion.Mood * 30;
        s += (int)emotion.Stress * 30 ;
        w += (int)emotion.Wellbeing * 30;
        c30++;
    }
    else
    {
        m += (int)emotion.Mood * 20;
        s += (int)emotion.Stress * 20;
        w += (int)emotion.Wellbeing * 20;
        c20++;
    }
}

// Final numbers
int c = 50 * c50 + 30 * c30 + 20 * c20;
m = m / c;
s = s /c;
w = w / c;
```

What About Android and iOS?

In Chapter 3, we discussed various libraries available for HealthVault. In particular, there are libraries available for Android (Java) and iOS (Objective-C) that allow a developer to implement a mobile application on these platforms. These libraries are open source and commercial-friendly.

We don't show the code for a sample application for these platforms, but the functionality available is very similar to the Windows Phone 7 library, and the material covered in this chapter will be equally useful.

The Android library is available with the HealthVault Java SDK on Codeplex, and the HealthVault iOS library is available on GitHub. It is left as an exercise to the reader to create solutions for these platforms.

Mobile Web Applications

Earlier in this chapter, we discussed the architectural choice to develop a client application for our Mood Tracker. However, web applications do have the choice to use the Web for delivery. In fact, we might want to link the Mood tracker application to our Quantified Self web application so that a user can see other relevant data in a web browser.

It's important to remember that a web application is a separate application entity from a native client application and that the user has to authorize it separately. The Quantified Self application, when launched from the Mood tracker, will ask the user to sign in and authorize it.

Web applications can use standard browser-detection techniques to present a mobile view of the content. HealthVault Shell does configure its view for mobile applications, and the calling application can always force a mobile view by adding *mobile=true* to the URL parameters. It would be a good exercise for the reader to implement a mobile view of the quantified self application.

Contributing to the Mood Tracker Application

The source for the Mood Tracker Windows Phone application is available at *http://enablingprogrammableself.com*, and we are inviting you, dear reader, to extend this application and make it your own. Perhaps fork the Git repository and contribute your code back, or create iOS and Android versions of it!

CHAPTER 6

The Last Mile: Releasing Applications to Users

*"Be careful about reading health books.
You may die of a misprint."*

—Mark Twain

Over the last few chapters we have gained an understanding of the HealthVault API (Chapter 3), learned about building a HealthVault web application with a focus on the HealthVault data types (Chapter 4), and built an engaging mobile application (Chapter 5). An application's life cycle typically involves testing the application, releasing it to the user, and then monitoring it for anomalies, tasks that entail special requirements in a HealthVault context. This chapter will highlight best practices for releasing, maintaining, and marketing HealthVault applications to end users.

Testing Your Application

Well-written software goes through multiple test cycles, including both automated and manual tests. This section outlines some valuable test scenarios around HealthVault account management, API interfaces, and data types, which you should consider in addition to other tests.

HealthVault enables people to share and manage multiple health records. In Chapter 3, we covered account management and ways to configure record switching. You need to ensure your application works with a HealthVault account that has multiple records. The best way to achieve this is to create several test accounts with multiple health records and try your application with them.

Another important aspect of account management is sharing. You can test this by sharing a HealthVault record with another person and then making sure that person can authenticate your application in association with that record. In case of insufficient permissions, your application should show an error message.

HealthVault provides an XML-based Web API. This API is accessible through programming libraries available through various HealthVault libraries and SDKs, as discussed in Chapter 3. While developing an application, you should pay special attention to any failure codes returned from HealthVault. In fact, make sure you log nonsuccess return codes from API calls to HealthVault so that you can investigate the reasons for failure. HealthVault provides a comprehensive list of status codes returned by the service at *http://msdn.microsoft.com/en-us/library/hh567902.aspx*. Particularly interesting is `CREDENTIAL_TOKEN_EXPIRED`, which your application should handle by requesting a new credentials token from HealthVault. The HealthVault .NET SDK and Mobile SDKs handle this status appropriately for you. In case you see the `INVALID_XML` status code, you should look closer at your request to make sure the XML is valid for various HealthVault methods and data type schemas, which are available at *http://developer .healthvault.com*.

HealthVault enables a coherent and well-adopted data ecosystem. It is very important to make sure that your application works well in this data ecosystem and uses the HealthVault data types appropriately. Chapter 4 explains HealthVault data types in detail. The best way to make sure you are reading a data type appropriately is to create a few instances of the type you are consuming with various possible permutations and combinations and then access them in your application. Get Real Consulting offers a great tool called HealthVault X-ray (*http://xray.getrealconsulting.com/*) that enables you to create myriad instances of the data type you are consuming in an appropriate test account.

The second aspect of working with the data types is to make sure that the information you are writing is consumable by other applications. The HealthVault team offers a tool called HealthVault Data Checkup at *http://datacheckup.healthvault-ppe.com/ hvappcheckup*. This tool works against data written by your application in a test record and finds any compatibility issues. Currently, the HealthVault Data Checkup tool supports only a limited number of types. Another mechanism to ensure that your application plays well in the HealthVault ecosystem is to copy your test records through HealthVault X-Ray in a production test account, authorize other HealthVault applications to access this account, and then confirm that the information is consumable by these applications.

Frequently, applications code properties of HealthVault data types improperly or are not able to parse a flexible date format as used in HealthVault. Review Chapter 4 to make sure you handle these cases.

Releasing Your Application to End Users

After testing your application thoroughly, including the conditions listed in the previous section, you are ready to release it to end users. The HealthVault team has documented the release process, termed the Go-Live Process, on the HealthVault Developer Center at *http://msdn.microsoft.com/en-us/healthvault/bb962148*.

The first step in this process it to ensure that you have signed a business agreement with HealthVault and have an identifier associated with your partner account. This is a nontechnical step and can be done long before your application is ready to be released.

Having established a partner account with Microsoft, you can submit a request to the technical team to review your application in the preproduction environment and push it to the HealthVault production environment. The review typically tests that your application plays well in the HealthVault ecosystem and uses the brand appropriately.

Once your application is available for the world to use, an important step is to network with fellow applications! This can be done using the wiki provided by the HealthVault team at *http://partners.mshealthcommunity.com/hv_eco/w/wiki/partner-directory.aspx*. In addition to business networking, this wiki is used by applications to notify the development community of any extensions to data types that they have implemented. Having well-documented extensions available makes it easy for other applications to work with data created by your application, giving you the benefit of network effects.

The last step in your Go-Live Process is to make sure that your application is discoverable to end users. This typically means working with the HealthVault team to become part of their application directory at *http://www.healthvault.com*.

Monitoring and Maintaining Your Application

Congratulations on getting that application out there! Whether you have created a client or a web application, it's very important to monitor its health.

You should log all the failed calls to the HealthVault web service. For additional debugging, the HealthVault SDK provides a tracing mechanism that you can use to log all the request responses. The mechanics of this are detailed at *http://msdn.microsoft .com/en-us/library/ff803626.aspx*. The HealthVault team monitors their development forums, available at *http://www.msdn.com/healthvault*, and you can use them to report any anomalies or failures in the service.

Each release of the HealthVault .NET SDK is supported for two years, and the team frequently adds enhancements and bug fixes to the newer releases. SDKs and libraries available in other language—Java, Python, etc.—are also updated by the community. As part of maintaining your application, you should make sure you monitor the underlying libraries so that you can upgrade your service to use the most robust offerings.

Another important aspect of maintaining a HealthVault application is to maintain its security artifacts, such as the application certificate and user tokens. HealthVault uses X509 certificates to authenticate web applications; you should make sure that the certificates you use for your application have the appropriate validity to function for a long time. HealthVault uses long-lived user tokens for client applications, and you should make sure that these applications frequently refresh the tokens.

Adding New Features to Your Application

Having a well-tested, well-maintained, and usable application will frequently result in a number of feature requests from users, which is not a bad problem to have! Many of these feature requests will necessitate support for additional HealthVault data types.

When you update your application to access new HealthVault data types, you must request the user to reauthorize your application so that it can access these additional data types. Another feature available from HealthVault is optional rules, which are data type authorization rules that ask permission only for additional data types. In addition to providing a smooth upgrade curve, optional rules also enable you to run an older version of your application side by side with the new version in case your users prefer not to upgrade. You can read more about optional rules at *http://msdn.microsoft.com/en-us/library/ff803609.aspx*.

Updating the data type rules of an application is not automatic, and an application typically needs to go through the HealthVault Go-Live process at *http://msdn.microsoft.com/en-us/healthvault/bb962148* to release updates in the HealthVault production environment.

Taking Your Application International!

Throughout this book, we have worked with HealthVault as it is available in United States. However, HealthVault has a growing list of implementation partners, and the platform is available in Canada, the UK, and Germany as of this writing. You can work with the HealthVault team to explore releasing your application in each of these countries.

The important aspect to keep in mind is that HealthVault as a service is completely globalized and internationalized. The request and response string that HealthVault displays to a user can be changed to appropriate locales. In fact, you can also make a Spanish version of your application available in the United States. The HealthVault Application Configuration Center, through its Localize tab, allows developers to configure their applications with Spanish strings so that when a user with Spanish browser settings accesses HealthVault, the application's authorization screen is shown with the appropriate language. The HealthVault Shell redirect interface, which is discussed in detail in Chapter 3, also respects an `lcid=Locale ID` parameter in its query string to show the appropriate display language in the user interface.

Additionally, HealthVault offers an internationalized set of units and time formats to allow applications to work with appropriate standards in the target country.

With this information, you are all set to stride into the exciting world of enabling Quantified Self with HealthVault!

Further Resources

This section highlights some important resource available for HealthVault development.

Need Reference Information?

The HealthVault MSDN site, *http://www.msdn.com/healthvault*, is a great resource on all things HealthVault. HealthVault features and SDK information is available in the reference section at *http://msdn.microsoft.com/en-us/library/aa155110.aspx*. The HealthVault team has an active blog at *http://blogs.msdn.com/b/healthvault/* and a list of frequently asked questions at *http://blogs.msdn.com/b/healthvaultfaq/*.

Have a Question?

The HealthVault Forums at *http://social.msdn.microsoft.com/forums/en-US/health vault/* are a great place to ask technical questions.

Development Tools

Fiddler (*http://fiddler2.com/fiddler2/*) is a great tool to enable request-response tracing for web applications. This tool will help you look at and analyze XML information being exchanged with the HealthVault platform.

Get Real Consulting's X-Ray for HealthVault (*https://xray.getrealconsulting.com/*) is an indispensable tool for HealthVault development. It offers the ability to create data in a HealthVault preproduction and production environment and to export and import information.

The HealthVault team hosts Developer Center tools at *http://developer.healthvault .com/*. This page is very handy for looking at HealthVault method and data type schemas.

HealthVault Application Data Checkup (*http://datacheckup.healthvault-ppe.com/ hvappcheckup*) offers lint functionality for data written by your application. This tool highlights best practices for writing data to HealthVault for a select set of data types.

Mapping Your Data to HealthVault

Chapter 4 summarizes the intent and use of various data types in HealthVault. Didier Thizy has a good post at *http://www.macadamian.com/insight/healthcare_detail/mapping_hl7_phm_to_healthvault/* on mapping the HL7 PHM standard to HealthVault.

The HealthVault team maintains a detailed mapping of the ASTM Continuity of Care Record standard to HealthVault data types on MSDN at *http://msdn.microsoft.com/en-us/healthvault/ee663895*. The reference article at *http://msdn.microsoft.com/en-us/library/ff803579.aspx* is a great resource for using CCR data in HealthVault.

About the Author

Vaibhav Bhandari is a seasoned software professional with several years of experience in technical development and management positions. He has led software development through multiple product cycles in varied businesses at Microsoft. His experience spans Windows PowerShell, Windows Mobile Operating System, and Microsoft Health-Vault. During the past three and a half years as part of the Microsoft HealthVault team, he has worked with developers and partners to design and implement health solutions on HealthVault. He has spoken and presented at several prestigious conferences including OSCON (2010 and 2011) and Health 2.0. He is active in the Healthcare IT community and shares an inside view on health technology with a popular blog. When not involved with healthcare and technology, he can be found mountaineering in the North Cascades near his home or off exploring faraway lands on his bicycle.

Get even more for your money.

Join the O'Reilly Community, and register the O'Reilly books you own. It's free, and you'll get:

- $4.99 ebook upgrade offer
- 40% upgrade offer on O'Reilly print books
- Membership discounts on books and events
- Free lifetime updates to ebooks and videos
- Multiple ebook formats, DRM FREE
- Participation in the O'Reilly community
- Newsletters
- Account management
- 100% Satisfaction Guarantee

Signing up is easy:

1. **Go to: oreilly.com/go/register**
2. **Create an O'Reilly login.**
3. **Provide your address.**
4. **Register your books.**

Note: English-language books only

To order books online:
oreilly.com/store

For questions about products or an order:
orders@oreilly.com

To sign up to get topic-specific email announcements and/or news about upcoming books, conferences, special offers, and new technologies:
elists@oreilly.com

For technical questions about book content:
booktech@oreilly.com

To submit new book proposals to our editors:
proposals@oreilly.com

O'Reilly books are available in multiple DRM-free ebook formats. For more information:
oreilly.com/ebooks

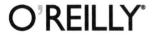

O'REILLY®

Spreading the knowledge of innovators | oreilly.com

The information you need, when and where you need it.

With Safari Books Online, you can:

Access the contents of thousands of technology and business books

- Quickly search over 7000 books and certification guides
- Download whole books or chapters in PDF format, at no extra cost, to print or read on the go
- Copy and paste code
- Save up to 35% on O'Reilly print books
- **New!** Access mobile-friendly books directly from cell phones and mobile devices

Stay up-to-date on emerging topics before the books are published

- Get on-demand access to evolving manuscripts.
- Interact directly with authors of upcoming books

Explore thousands of hours of video on technology and design topics

- Learn from expert video tutorials
- Watch and replay recorded conference sessions

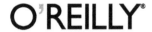

Spreading the knowledge of innovators   safari.oreilly.com

Lightning Source UK Ltd.
Milton Keynes UK
UKHW031054070222
398311UK00005B/164